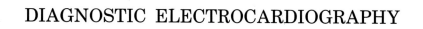

DIAGNOSTIC ELECTROCARDIOGRAPHY

DIAGNOSTIC ELECTROCARDIOGRAPHY

WITHDRAWN

MICHAEL C. RITOTA, M.D., D.SC. (*h.c.*), F.A.C.P.

Director, Department of Medicine, Columbus Hospital, Newark
Attending in Medicine, Saint Michael's Hospital, Newark

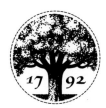

J. B. LIPPINCOTT COMPANY

Philadelphia and Toronto

ISBN 0-397-50246-X

Library of Congress Catalog Card Number 68-26656

Printed in the United States of America

9 8

Preface

Cardiovascular diseases cause more than half of all deaths in the United States—indeed, acute coronary thrombosis or acute myocardial infarction has been called the "twentieth century epidemic." In addition, of patients seen by the general practitioner, as many as 50 per cent are found to have cardiac symptoms or actually to be suffering from heart disease.

Heart disease can be aggravated or caused by other diseases. Conversely, heart disease may precipitate diseases of organs such as the brain, as well as the kidney, liver and other visceral organs that depend on cardiac output for proper function.

It is therefore important that physicians in general practice and in specialties other than cardiology be able to interpret cardiac symptoms correctly, since this ability will be useful both in differential diagnosis and in revealing relationships between these symptoms and disorders in other organs and systems.

Electrocardiography is today increasingly important as a tool in the diagnosis of heart disease. It is important to every general physician and specialist, and to interns and nurses connected with cardiovascular services. Knowledge of electrocardiography aids both physicians and students in the evaluation of the treatment and management—and, therefore, of the prognosis—of heart disease.

The purpose of this book is to present simply and accurately the basic knowledge essential to the interpretation of commonly seen electrocardiograms. To accomplish this with the greatest brevity and clarity, the text is organized in outline form, and, since a picture is worth ten thousand words, diagrams and actual ECGs are used to illustrate each point discussed and every feature of the ECG of diagnostic value. Each type of ECG is first presented diagrammatically and much enlarged, for ease of visualization of the features characteristic of that type. The text calls attention to features of diagnostic significance and also to associated conditions. The normal cycle and its components (P–Q–R–S–T–U waves) are stressed in the earlier chapters; the abnormal patterns are shown in the later chapters.

It is hoped that this book will be valuable not only to interns, residents and nurses in Intensive Coronary Care Units but also to all practitioners interested in electrocardiography.

MICHAEL C. RITOTA

Acknowledgment

Acknowledgment is due primarily to the general practitioner, whose service is unceasing and of inestimable value in the endless war against disease.

I wish, next, to express my great admiration of the teachers responsible in large measure for my education in cardiology and electrocardiography: Dr. Sidney P. Schwartz, Dr. Emanuel Goldberger, Dr. Abraham Jezer, the late Dr. J. B. Schwedel, Dr. Scott Butterworth, Dr. William B. Hitzig, Dr. Ralph Miller, Dr. Leonard Dreifus, Dr. Joseph Riseman, Dr. Harry Gross and Dr. H. J. Marriott.

I sincerely appreciate the opportunity given me by Saint Michael's Hospital and Columbus Hospital to teach electrocardiography to physicians in New Jersey, whose inspiration and encouragement moved the author to the writing of this book.

To Mr. Harold Scholl and my son Theodore Ritota, a medical student at the University of Autonoma Medical School, Guadalajara, Mexico, I am grateful for the diagrams and other illustrations used in this book.

I am deeply indebted to my friend and teacher, Dr. Ralph Miller, who has patiently and meticulously criticized the text.

Finally, I wish to thank Mr. J. Brooks Stewart for his patient assistance and cooperation in the preparation of this book.

Contents

1. TECHNICAL AND MECHANICAL CONSIDERATIONS. 1
   Standardization of the Electrocardiogram 1
   Marking Code 2
   Indications for Taking an Electrocardiogram 2
   Artifacts in the Electrocardiogram 4

2. P–Q–R–S–T–U CYCLE 5
   The P Wave. 6
   The P–R Interval. 7
   The Q Wave 8
   QRS Complex. 9
   The S–T Segment 11
   The T Wave. 13
   The U Wave 16
   The Q–T Interval 19
   Determination of Cardiac Rate. 19

3. PLOTTING THE ELECTRICAL AXIS 22
   Five Basic Patterns 22
   Origin and Development of the Triaxial and Hexaxial Systems 23
   Axis Deviation 24
   Methods for Determining Axis Deviation 25

4. SINUS RHYTHMS, SINUS ARRHYTHMIAS, AND ATRIAL RHYTHMS 29
   Sinus Rhythm and Sinus Arrhythmias. 29
     Sinus Rhythm 29
     Sinus Arrhythmia. 29
     Sinus Bradycardia. 33

4. SINUS RHYTHMS, SINUS ARRHYTHMIAS, AND ATRIAL RHYTHMS—*(Cont.)*

  Sinus Tachycardia 37
  The More Common Atrial Arrhythmias 38
  Atrial Extrasystoles 40
  Atrial Tachycardia 43
  Atrial Flutter 47
  Atrial Fibrillation 49

5. PREMATURE VENTRICULAR SYSTOLES 56

6. BUNDLE BRANCH BLOCK 60
  Conditions Associated With Left or Right Bundle Branch Block 60
  Complete Left Bundle Branch Block 69
  Complete Right Bundle Branch Block 69

7. VENTRICULAR HYPERTROPHY 70
  Left Ventricular Hypertrophy 70
  Right Ventricular Hypertrophy 71

8. NODAL RHYTHM 82

9. HEART BLOCK 88
  First Degree Heart Block 88
  Second Degree Atrioventricular Block 88
  Complete Heart Block (Third Degree A–V Block) 91

10. ACUTE PERICARDITIS 95

11. MYOCARDIAL INFARCTION 101
  Recognizing the Candidate for Coronary Heart Disease 101

11.   MYOCARDIAL INFARCTION — (*Cont.*)
        Epidemiology of Myocardial Infarction 101
        The Predisposed Candidate 101
        Etiology of Myocardial Infarction 101
        Anatomic Factors 101
        Pathologic Changes 101
        Signs and Symptoms of Myocardial Infarction 102
        Cardiac Serum Enzymes 102
        Electrocardiographic Criteria in Myocardial Infarction 102
        The Electrocardiogram in the Diagnosis of Myocardial Infarction 105

12.   ANGINA PECTORIS 118

13.   THE MASTER'S-ROSENFELD TEST 119

14.   CARDIOPULMONARY DISEASE: COR PULMONALE, ACUTE, AND CHRONIC 125

15.   DIGITALIS AND THE ELECTROCARDIOGRAM 130

16.   ELECTROLYTES AND THE ELECTROCARDIOGRAM 139
        Hyperkalemia 139
        Hypokalemia 139
        Hypercalcemia 139
        Hypocalcemia 139

17.   VENTRICULAR TACHYCARDIA — VENTRICULAR FLUTTER — VENTRICULAR FIBRILLA-
        TION — CARDIAC ARREST 148
        Ventricular Tachycardia 148
        Ventricular Flutter 157
        Ventricular Fibrillation 158
        Cardiac Arrest 160

INDEX 167

History of the Electrocardiogram

The electrocardiograph, recording the minute electrical currents from the heart, is an achievement of the highest order in medical technology. It is a "biophysical machine" furnishing data that are highly reliable and among the most accurate that may be obtained.

Experiments in animal electricity were first performed by Luigi Galvani (1737-1798), the famous professor of anatomy at the University of Bologna, who hypothesized that the twitching of a frog's muscles which were pierced with metal was due to an electrical current. This concept of electrical impulses in muscle opened the way for progressive research in electrical energy and conduction in the tissues of the heart.

The earliest records of electrical activity of the heart were made in 1878, with the recording wires connected directly to the heart.

In 1887, Augustus D. Waller developed a method whereby electrical currents in the living heart could be recorded at the surface of the body and measured indirectly. This was done by running lead wires from a capillary electrometer and recording and measuring the shadow of its oscillation.

William Einthoven, the great Dutch physiologist, in 1901 invented the string galvanometer. The string galvanometer consists of a fine quartz string covered with gold or silver and suspended between the poles of a powerful electromagnet. The small current (measured in millivolts) passing through the string sets up a magnetic field, causing a deflection of the string. The shadow of the string and of this deflection is cast by a strong beam of light directed through apertures in the arms of the magnet and is magnified by lenses similar in arrangement to that of a microscope. The images of these deflections are focused on photographic plate or film moving at the desired speed.

Within the last ten or fifteen years machinery has been developed with amplifying tubes capable of magnifying this "current deflection" 3,000 times. An electrically heated stylus transposes the changes onto waxed paper.

The string galvanometer was comparatively difficult to manage, and the film had to be developed, with consequent delay in the availability of the information, whereas the presently used equipment has a direct writing stylus and can be read from moment to moment. Originally, only three leads were used; at present, twelve leads are used in the conventional electrocardiogram.

More compact machines are being made and new applications are being found. High fidelity electrocardiographs depict minute changes in the electrocardiogram; and radio-cardiography is now being used with stress tests, both in terrestrial settings and in investigations relating to man's activities in space.

DIAGNOSTIC ELECTROCARDIOGRAPHY

CHAPTER 1

Technical and Mechanical Considerations

Standardization of the Electrocardiogram

For the electrocardiogram to be technically accurate certain conditions must be met. The essential prerequisites for good tracings with a minimum of technical errors are:
1. Proper standardization
2. Proper positioning of extremity and chest leads
3. Proper coding

There Must Be Proper Standardization of One Millivolt (Fig. 1-1).

The horizontal lines on the electrocardiograph paper are spaced 1 millimeter apart and are used to measure voltage. The 1-cm. standardization is the normal standardization. It is used universally so that comparative studies of tracings can be made readily. Standardization of 0.5 cm. is used when there is high voltage or the amplitude of the complexes exceeds the size of the paper. When the stylus inscribes above and beyond the limits of the paper, the complexes can be seen better by reducing the voltage to $\frac{1}{2}$ cm. Double the amplitudes obtained at 0.5 cm. will give the values for 1-cm. standardization. A 2-cm. standardization is used to increase the amplitude of fibrillatory ("f") waves, flutter ("F") waves, low P waves, and other such waves that may be difficult to discern at 1 cm. because of their miniature amplitudes.

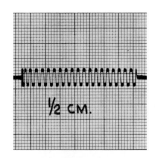

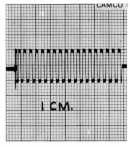

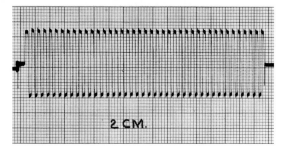

FIG. 1-1. Standardization of 1 millivolt. (*Top*) At 0.5 cm. (5 mm.) $\frac{1}{2}$ mv. (*Center*) At 1 cm. (10 mm.) 1 mv. (*Bottom*) At 2 cm. (20 mm.) 2 mv.

There Must Be a Constant Standard Positioning of the Precordial Electrodes and the Standard Leads (Fig. 1-2).

The lead tips of the lead cable are designated as follows:
RA (right arm)
LA (left arm)
LL (left leg)
RL (right leg)
RL is the grounding wire; the other leads form the Einthoven triangle (Fig. 1-3). The leads must be placed correctly; abnormal patterns result from wrong positioning.

The precordial leads are positioned from V_1 to V_6 (Fig. 1-4) by the use of a small suction cup on lead P (precordial—or C, chest). Lack of precision in location of these leads will result in variation in the patterns. This becomes especially important if serial electrocardiograms are taken or electrocardiograms are taken by different technicians at different times or places. Therefore all rules must be standardized.

There Must Be Careful Code Marking of Each Individual Lead, as Described Below.

Code marking should be done as the electrocardiogram is being taken, in order to avoid errors later, in the mounting of the tracing and lead identification. Coding is best represented by dots (or very short dashes which simulate dots) and long dashes. The code given here is in general use. However, any method is acceptable so long as it is simple and clear. If any code other than the one shown is used, the explanation should be noted on the E.C.G. as soon as the lead is transcribed.

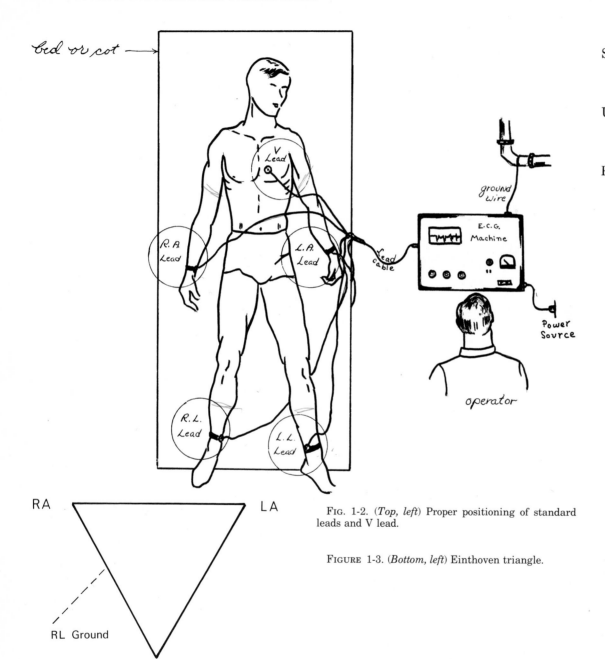

FIG. 1-2. (*Top, left*) Proper positioning of standard leads and V lead.

FIGURE 1-3. (*Bottom, left*) Einthoven triangle.

Marking Code

STANDARD LEADS	CODE
Lead I (left arm–right arm)	•
Lead II (left leg–right arm)	••
Lead III (left arm–left leg)	•••
UNIPOLAR (AUGMENTED) LEADS	
aVR (right arm)	—
aVL (left arm)	— —
aVF (left leg)	— — —
PRECORDIAL LEADS	
V_1	— •
V_2	— ••
V_3	— •••
V_4	— ••••
V_5	— •••••
V_6	— ••••••
V_3R	— ••• —
V_4R	— •••• —

Indications for Taking an Electrocardiogram

1. Severe chest pain
   A good motto to follow is: "Any pain above the diaphragm, take an electrocardiogram."
2. Sudden onset of dyspnea
3. Any tachycardia, bradycardia, or arrhythmia
4. Shock state
5. Syncope
6. Postoperative hypotension
7. Coma
8. All murmurs
9. Cardiomegaly
10. Severe right upper quadrant (gallbladder (?)) *or* epigastric (ulcer (?)) pain
11. Congenital *or* acquired cyanosis
12. Daily cardiac monitoring in coronary intensive care units
13. Trauma to the chest
14. Preoperatively, for patients over 50 years of age
15. All cases of hypertension

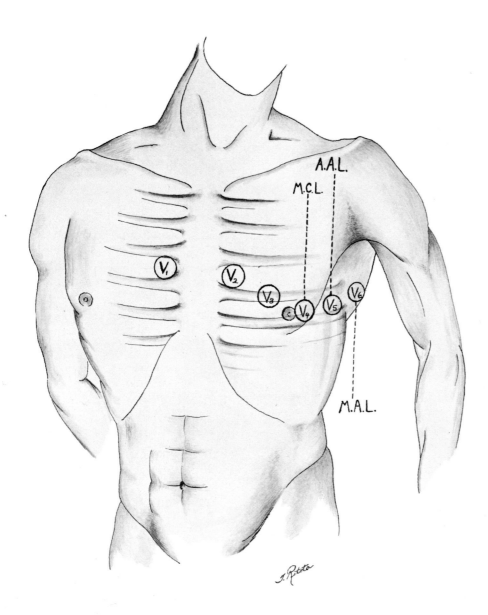

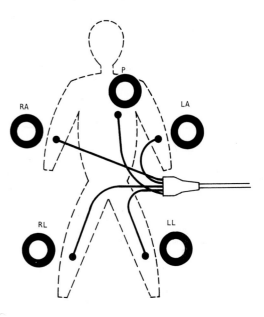

FIG. 1-5. Procedure for taking the electrocardiogram.
1. Connect power cord.
2. Set lead selector to 0.
3. Apply jelly and electrodes to patient.
4. Turn power switch on, set polarity.
5. Attach patient cable.
6. Position stylus to center of chart.
7. Push *Standardize* button to check sensitivity.
8. Record EKG:
   (a) Set lead selector to 1 and turn on record switch.
   (b) Without stopping chart, move lead selector to 2.
   (c) Record lead 3, aVr, aVl, and aVf in same manner.
   (d) Turn lead selector to dot between aVf and V. Stop recording. Prepare electrode positions on patient's chest.
   (e) Attach vactrode, move lead selector to V. Turn on recorder.
   (f) Proceed as in Step (c) for the other V positions. Always set lead selector to dot before or after V when removing vactrode.
   (g) Move lead selector to CF and turn on recorder.
   (h) Stop recording and move lead selector to 0.
9. Turn off power switch.
(Courtesy of Cambridge Instrument Co., Ossining, N. Y.)

FIG. 1-4. The landmarks for the precordial leads (V leads)
V_1 — 4th interspace at the right border of the sternum
V_2 — 4th interspace at the left border of the sternum
V_3 — left parasternal line midway between V_2 and V_4
V_4 — 5th interspace in the left midclavicular line
V_5 — in the anterior axillary line at the level of V_4
V_6 — in the midaxillary line at the level of V_4 and V_5
MCL — Midclavicular line. AAL — Anterior axillary line. MAL — Midaxillary line.

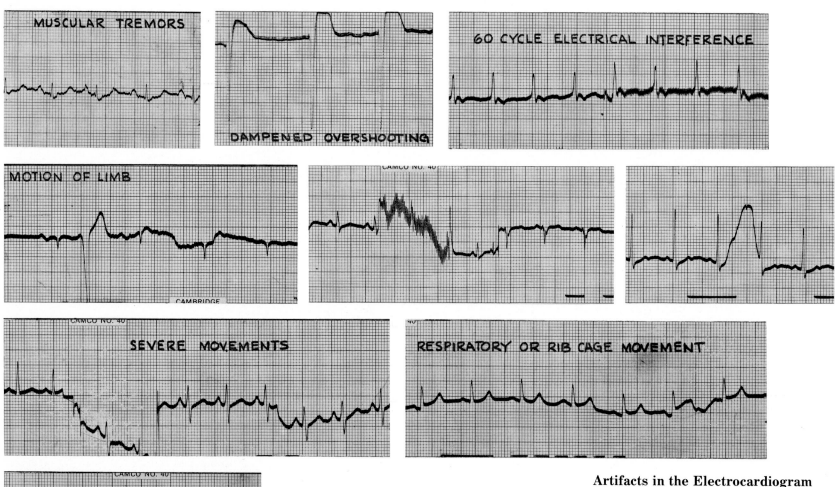

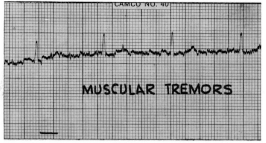

Fig. 1-6. Artifacts found in cardiogram tracings. *Second row, (Center)* Motion and electrical interference. *(Right)* Motion of limb. "Dampened overshooting" indicates that the stylus is hitting the limits of its excursion.

Artifacts in the Electrocardiogram

Artifacts seen in tracings are frequently the result of technical errors and may be due to (a) electrical interference; (b) loose lead wire connections; (c) poor application of jelly or other contact substance. Artifacts may also be caused by (a) motion of the patient, (b) muscle tremor, and (c) severe nervous disorders of the muscular system.

CHAPTER 2

P-Q-R-S-T-U Cycle

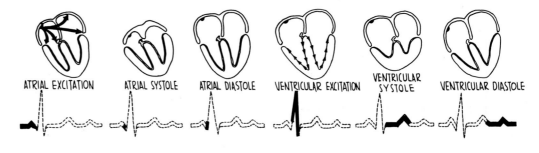

Atrial excitation starts at the sino-auricular node and spreads through both atria. The excitation starts at some point before the P wave and includes the entire P wave. The P wave represents depolarization of the atria.

The P-R segment is the period of atrial repolarization.

The Q wave represents the first wave of ventricular excitation or depolarization.

The P-R interval is the summation of the periods of atrial depolarization and atrial repolarization.

The QRS interval represents the complete depolarization of the ventricular musculature.

The S-T segment represents the early phase of repolarization. The S-T segment and the T wave together represent almost all of the complete phase of ventricular repolarization. The Q-T interval represents the time of ventricular activation or depolarization through the period of repolarization.

Ventricular diastole follows the end of the T wave.

The U wave represents the after potential of the T wave. This is in the recovery phase and during ventricular diastole.

"J" indicates the junction between the QRS complex and the S-T segment.

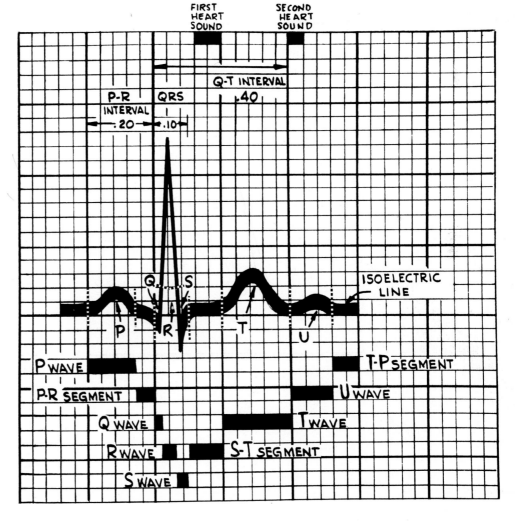

Fig. 2-1. (*Right*) P-Q-R-S-T-U cycle.

The P Wave

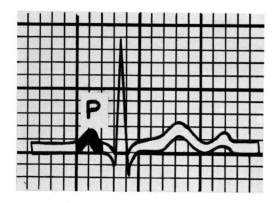

FIGURE 2-2

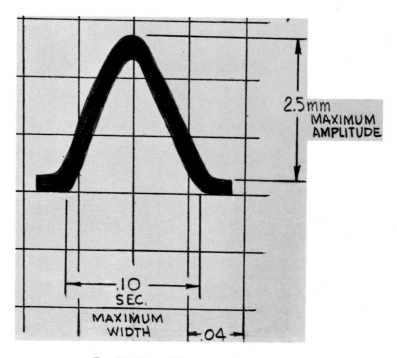

FIG. 2-3. Normal P wave: maximum limits.

One of the most important features of the ECG record is the P wave. The rate—or the absence—of P waves helps to establish rhythm and is important in the recognition of most arrhythmias. In addition to rhythm and rate, diagnostically significant characteristics of the P wave are size, shape and relationship to the QRS.

"Cherchez le P"—search for the P wave— is a good rule to follow.

The P wave is the initial upward deflection in leads I, II, and III and represents atrial excitation, or depolarization.

The P wave is largest in lead II.

The Normal P Wave (Fig. 2-3)

The normal P wave is usually upright in leads I and II and may be flat, diphasic or inverted in lead III. It is upright in aVL and aVF and inverted in aVR. In the precordial leads the P may be inverted in V_1 and V_2 and upright in V_3 to V_6. It is seldom taller than 2.5 mm. Its width does not exceed 0.10 sec. (see Fig. 2-3).

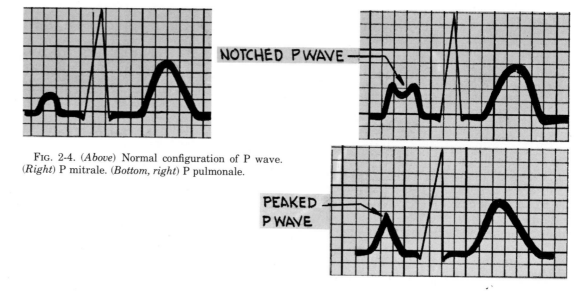

FIG. 2-4. (*Above*) Normal configuration of P wave. (*Right*) P mitrale. (*Bottom, right*) P pulmonale.

P-Wave Forms (Fig. 2-4).

Contrast the form of the normal P wave with the P mitrale and the P pulmonale.

P mitrale is bifid and usually is more than 0.10 sec. in width. The width of the notch (between its peaks) is at least 0.03 sec. P mitrale commonly is found in rheumatic heart disease with mitral stenosis; atrial septal defect; and tetralogy of Fallot.*

P pulmonale is seen most often in chronic emphysema, cor pulmonale and right ventricular hypertrophy. The P wave is sharply peaked and symmetrical in leads II, III and aVF. It is usually tall and prominent, but its measurements may be within normal limits.

*Thomas, P., and Dejong, D.: Brit. Heart J., 16:241, 1954.

The P-R Interval

The P-R interval measures the period of time from the beginning of the ascending limb of the P wave to the beginning of the Q wave or the R wave if no Q wave is formed. P-Q is equivalent to the P-R interval (Fig. 2-7).

The normal range of the P-R interval is 0.12 sec. to 0.20 or 0.21 sec. Any prolongation of the P-R interval denotes delay in atrioventricular nodal conduction. A prolonged P-R interval is first-degree heart block (Fig. 2-6).

The P-R interval varies with heart rate. The higher the rate the shorter the conduction time through the atria and the atrioventricular node to the bundle of His.

THE P-R INTERVAL AND THE HEART RATE*

HEART RATE (per min.)	P-R INTERVAL (in seconds)
40 to 70	0.20 to 0.21
71 to 90	0.19 to 0.20
91 to 120	0.18 to 0.19
121 to 140	0.17 to 0.18
141 to 160	0.16 to 0.17

* After Ashman and Hull: Essentials of Electrocardiography. New York, Macmillan, 1937.

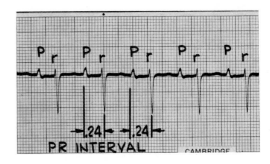

FIG. 2-6. Prolonged P-R interval in first-degree heart block. The P-R intervals marked (arrows) measure 0.24 seconds. The P-R interval here starts from the beginning of the P wave and ends at the onset of the ascending limb of the R wave.

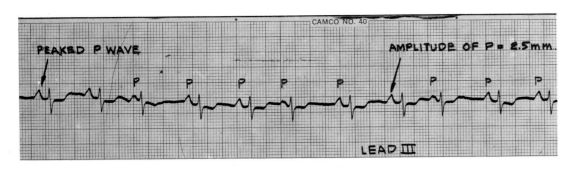

FIG. 2-5. (*Top*) Peaked P waves, cor pulmonale. The patient had chronic asthma and bronchitis. (*Bottom*) P mitrale. Large atrium. P waves are broader than 0.10 sec.

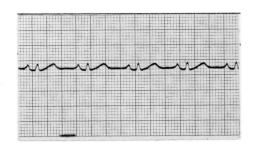

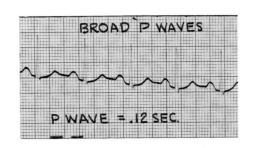

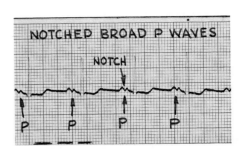

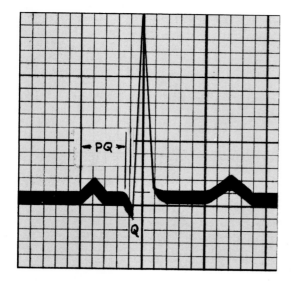

FIG. 2-7. The P-R interval. (*Left*) The P-R interval is measured from the beginning of the P wave to the beginning of the deflection of the Q wave (the first element of the QRS complex to appear). (*Right*) The P-R interval is measured from the beginning of the P wave to the junction of the P-R segment with the R wave. In this pattern no Q wave is written.

The Q Wave

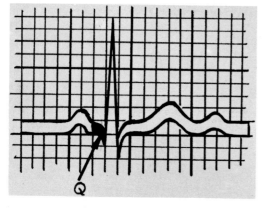

FIG. 2-8. The Q wave, normal configuration.

The Q wave is the first downward deflection following the P wave (Fig. 2-8).

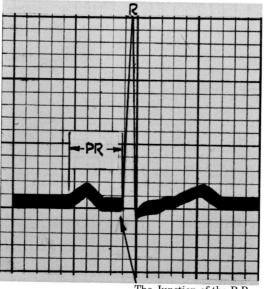

The Junction of the P-R Segment with R wave.

The width of the Q wave normally is less than 0.04 sec.

The amplitude of the Q wave is normal
in lead I when Q is less than 15% of R_1
in lead II when Q is less than 20% of R_2
in lead III when Q is less than 25% of R_3
In Figure 2-9 A, the Q wave is normal in respect to both width and depth. A Q wave may be normal in depth but abnormal in width (Fig. 2-9 B, Q is 0.04 sec. wide); it may be normal in width but abnormal in depth (Fig. 2-9 C); it may be abnormal in respect to both width and depth (Fig. 2-9 D).

QS Patterns.

QS deflections may be 0.06 to 0.08 sec. wide (Fig. 2-9 E). They are found normally in V_1 and V_2 and, possibly, in V_3. The QS pattern is also found normally in lead III and in aVR, aVL and aVF. It is found nor-

mally in aVR because this is normally a negative lead; it is found normally in aVL and aVF in vertical or transverse hearts by virtue of their position.

Through and through infarction (transmural) will produce a QS pattern in the lead facing the dead muscle (an "electrical window looking into the left ventricular cavity").

Vestigial Q Wave.

This wave is less than 0.03 sec. wide (Fig. 2-9 F). It appears in 30 per cent of old healed infarcts with patterns that have returned to normal and had no Q wave recorded in pre-infarction cardiograms. In left bundle branch block patterns, vestigial Q wave may be found in lead I and aVL, or in V_5, V_6, signifying an infarction.

FIG. 2-9. (*A-F*) Types of Q waves.

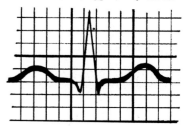

A. Normal Q wave, in both width (less than 0.04 sec.) and depth.

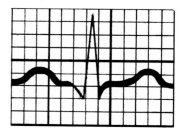

B. Wide Q wave, with normal depth. (*Continued on facing page.*)

FIGURE 2-9 (Cont.)

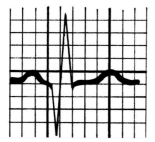

C. Deep Q wave, with normal width.

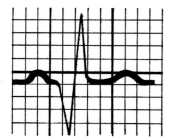

D. Wide and deep Q wave.

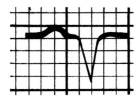

E. QS pattern (0.06 to 0.07 sec.).

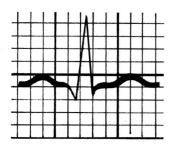

F. Vestigial Q wave (0.03 sec.).

QRS Complex

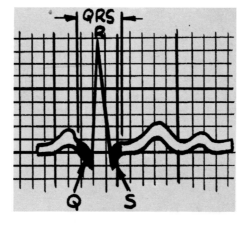

FIG. 2-10. The QRS complex. The QRS interval is measured from the beginning of the Q wave to the end of the S wave.

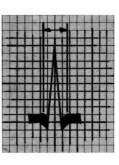

qRs pattern (0.12 sec.)

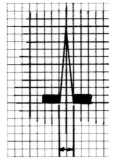

R pattern (0.08 sec.)

FIG. 2-11. How to measure QRS interval with various QRS patterns. Limit of arrows indicates QRS interval.

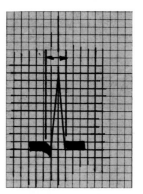

qR pattern (0.11 sec.)

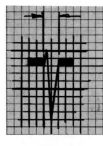

rS pattern (0.08 sec.)

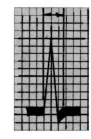

Rs pattern (0.11 sec.)

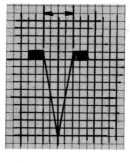

Qs pattern (0.16 sec.)

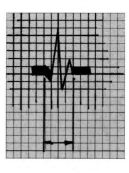

Rsr' pattern (0.16 sec.)

The QRS complex records the depolarization of the ventricular musculature and describes the massive electrical architecture of the ventricular conduction system. The QRS interval is the time required for complete depolarization and is measured from the onset of the Q wave, or of the R wave if no Q is written, to the end of the S wave or of the R wave if no S is written (Fig. 2-10). The QRS interval is measured in the lead in which it is the longest.

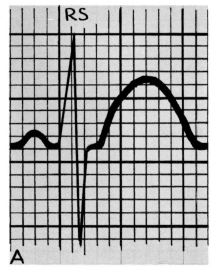

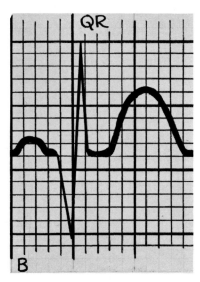

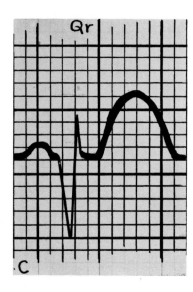

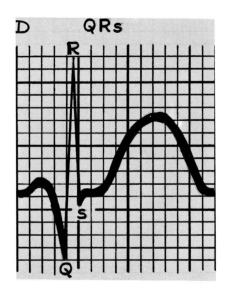

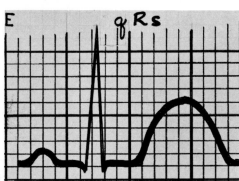

Fig. 2-12. QRS patterns.

A. The RS pattern is seen most commonly over the interventricular septum and is called the transitional zone pattern.

B. The QR pattern denotes a cavity potential or an electrical window with a substantial amount of myocardium remaining alive and electrically active in the area of the infarct to give a large positive deflection.

C. The Qr pattern is a cavity potential or an electrical window; the r indicates a small mass of active myocardium.

D. The QRs pattern is seen most commonly in infarction when there is a small electrical window with a substantial amount of myocardium.

E. The qRs pattern. This is the normal pattern. Note that the q is very small and the s is very small.

F. The qRS pattern may be a normal pattern. Note, however, that the q is small in width and depth, the R is tall and the S is deep and wide.

G. The qR pattern. The S wave is absent. This pattern is found over the left ventricle in normal beats.

H. The qRS pattern. This is found in V_5 and V_6 and in incomplete right bundle branch block.

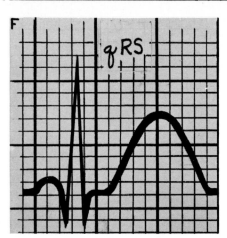

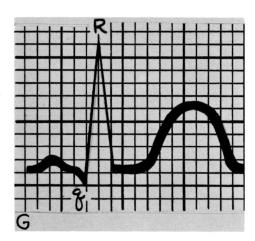

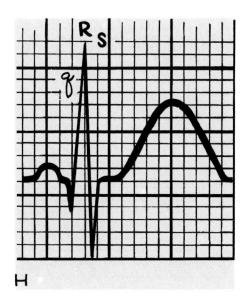

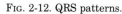

The upper limit of normal for QRS interval is 0.10 sec. A QRS interval of between 0.10 sec. and 0.12 sec. is indicative of incomplete bundle branch block. A QRS time of 0.12 sec. or more is usually associated with complete bundle branch block and is considered diagnostic.

Prolonged QRS is seen also in the following arrhythmias:

Ventricular extrasystole
Ventricular tachycardia
Aberrant ventricular conduction

QRS Patterns

Ventricular patterns may consist of the Q, R, and S waves, or of Q and R, R and S, or R alone. Capital letters are used to denote large amplitudes; small letters are used for waves of small amplitude.

Amplitude is measured in positive deflections from the top of the base line to the top of the R wave; in negative deflections S waves are measured from the bottom of the base line to the bottom of the deflection.

The S-T Segment

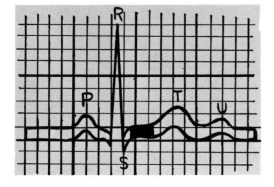

Fig. 2-13. The S-T segment.

The S-T segment represents the time interval from the end of the QRS interval to the onset of the T wave. It may also repre-

TABLE 2-1. NORMAL LIMITS OF S-T SEGMENTS AND T WAVES

LEAD	S-T DISPLACEMENT	AMPLITUDE OF T
I	+1 to −1 mm.	+1 mm. to +5 mm.
II	+1 to −1 mm.	+1 mm. to +5 mm.
III	+1 to −1 mm.	+1 mm. to +5 mm. May be upright, flat, diphasic, or inverted normally.
aVR	+1 to −1 mm.	Normal limits −1 to −6 mm. (inverted T wave) Positive T waves are abnormal.
aVL	+1 to −1 mm.	If the R wave is taller than 5 mm., then the T wave is abnormal if negative. If R is less than 5 mm., a negative T is normal.
aVF	+1 to −1 mm.	+5 to −1 mm.
V₁, V₂,	+2 to +4 mm. to −1 mm.	+5 to −4 mm.
V₃, V₄, V₅, V₆	+2 to +4 mm. to −1 mm.	+1 mm. to +13 mm.

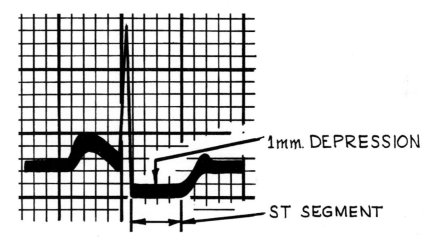

Fig. 2-14. A. Horizontal S-T segments. (*Cont. on p. 12*)

sent the time interval from the end of the R wave to the T wave when the S wave is absent. This interval physiologically represents the early phase of ventricular repolarization. The isoelectric line is the zero potential line—the interval between the T wave or U wave and the P wave. This interval is called the T-P interval. Physiologically it represents complete cardiac rest, or electrical inactivity.

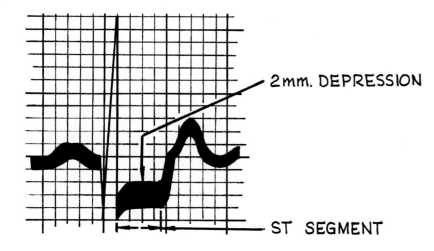

2mm. DEPRESSION

ST SEGMENT

FIGURE 2-14 B

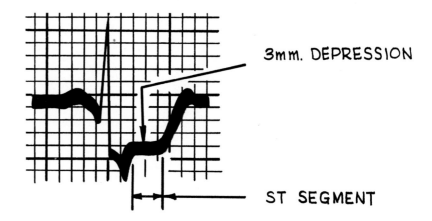

3mm. DEPRESSION

ST SEGMENT

FIGURE 2-14 C

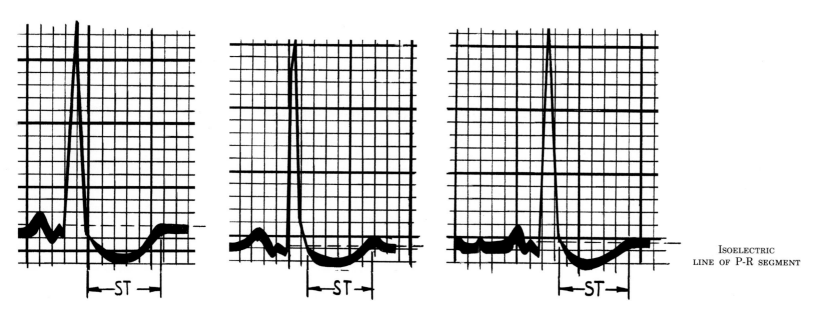

ST

ST

ST

ISOELECTRIC
LINE OF P-R SEGMENT

FIG. 2-15. S-T segments showing sagging depression. (*Left*) Concavity of the S-T segment is more than 1 mm., measured below the isoelectric line (dotted line) of the P-R segment. (*Center*) The S-T depression at its nadir (the lowest point) is 1 mm. below the P-R segment line. (*Right*) The concavity of the S-T segment at the nadir is at least 2 mm. in depth.

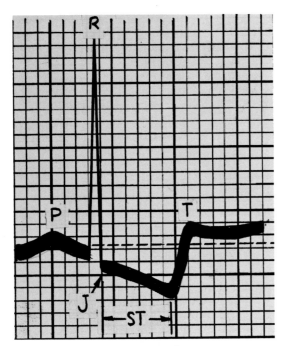

FIGURE 2-16 A

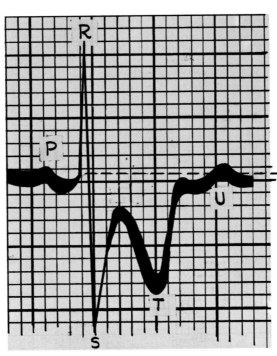

FIGURE 2-16 B

FIG. 2-16. S-T segments, showing angular depression. A. The S-T segment is depressed 1 mm. The T wave has been pulled down by the S-T segment. The S-T segment lies at an angle and below the base line. Therefore it shows angular depression. B. The entire S-T segment and the T wave have been pulled down 2.5 mm. below the P-R segment. The S-T segment is again angular and below the base line (isoelectric line). This is angular depression. (The dotted lines in A and B indicate the isoelectric line of the P-R segment.)

A rise of the S-T segment of more than one millimeter above the isoelectric line indicates abnormal S-T elevation.

A depression of the S-T segment of one millimeter or more indicates abnormal S-T depression.

Upward abnormalities indicate:

Infarction

Pericarditis

Ischemia

Normal S-T variation

Depression of S-T segment may be found in:

Ischemia

Digitalis effect

Right ventricular hypertrophy

Complete bundle branch block

An S-T segment that is flat or horizontal and longer than 0.08 or 0.12 second raises suspicion of ischemia.

There are 3 common types of ST depression.

1. Horizontal
2. Sagging
3. Angular

S-T segment variations indicative of ischemia are illustrated in Figures 2-14 to 2-16.

The T Wave

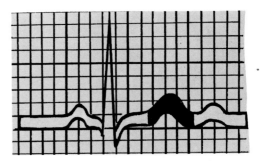

FIG. 2-17. The T wave.

The T wave is the first major upward deflection following the R wave. It represents the final phase of repolarization of the myocardium.

T waves may be abnormal in:

1. Amplitude
2. Shape
3. Polarity (direction)

Characteristic T Waves

Standard Leads	T Wave
Lead I	always positive
Lead II	always positive
Lead III	may be positive, flat or negative

Augmented Unipolar Leads	
aVR	always negative
aVL	usually positive; may be negative. Negative T wave is abnormal when the R wave is greater than 5 mm. in amplitude: associated with lateral wall infarction, ischemia or strain

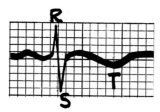

Normal T wave

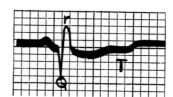

Cove plane T wave

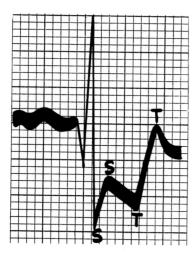

Ischemic T wave

aVF   almost always positive and upright; may be negative in horizontal heart. Otherwise, negative T wave is

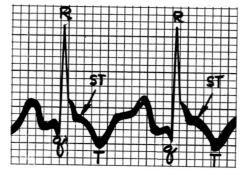

Negative T wave, sub-acute infarction

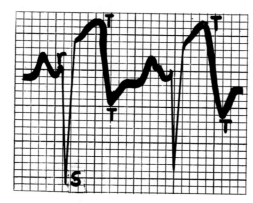

Negative chronic infarction T wave

ST-T elevation

Fig. 2-18. (*Continued on facing page.*)

evidence of posterior wall infarction, pulmonary embolism or right ventricular strain.

Precordial Leads

V_1 negative normally in 80% of patients
V_2 negative normally in 20% of patients
V_3 upright; amplitude, to 13 mm. (maximum)
V_4 upright; amplitude, to 13 mm. (maximum)
V_5 upright; amplitude, to 13 mm. (maximum)
V_6 upright; amplitude, to 13 mm. (maximum)

If deflection is more than 1 mm. in any of the precordial leads, the T wave is abnormal.

If amplitude of an upright T wave is less than 1 mm. in any of the standard and precordial leads, the T wave is abnormal.

Abnormal inverted T waves are found in the following conditions:

1. Myocardial ischemia
2. Ventricular hypertrophy
3. Complete bundle branch block (right or left)
4. Pericarditis
5. Cor pulmonale
6. Myocarditis and other myocardiopathies
7. Electrolyte imbalance
8. Metabolic diseases
9. Vitamin deficiency
10. Digitalis intoxication; other drugs having similar effects include quinidine and procainamide.
11. Acute or chronic myocardial infarction

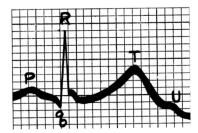

Normal T wave

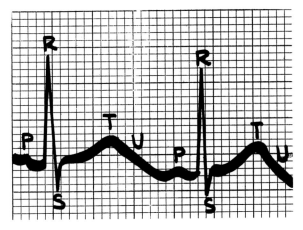

T-U fusion

FIGURE 2-18. (*Cont.*)

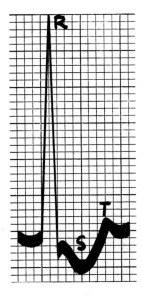

Digitalis T wave

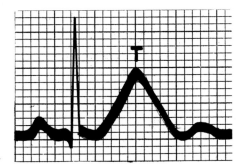

Broad peaked T wave

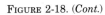

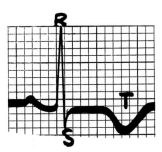

Chronic coronary T wave

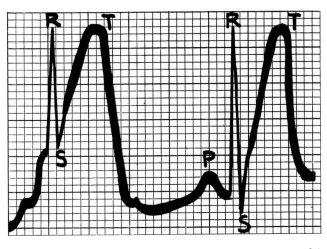

Giant peaked T waves (acute anterior wall infarction, very early)

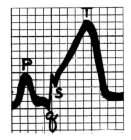

Acute infarction—
acute ST-elevation

Large T Waves

Negative Large T Waves*

CHARACTERISTICS

Found primarily in precordial leads, especially V_4 to V_6 (pathological)

Amplitude

As much as −28 mm. (negative T) has been reported.

Duration

Usually prolonged: Q-T duration increased by 25% to 100%

Regression

Usually a decrease in size over a period of days to months

Temporary improvement has been reported with

nitroglycerin

oxygen

papaverine

aminophylline

CONDITIONS IN WHICH LARGE NEGATIVE T WAVES ARE FOUND

Myocardial infarction

Subendocardial infarction

Subepicardial ischemia

Cerebrovascular accidents

Post-tachycardia syndrome

Positive Large T Waves†

CHARACTERISTICS

Found primarily in the precordial leads

Amplitude

Greater than 13 mm. in the precordial leads (abnormal)

Duration (Q-T interval)

Not necessarily prolonged, with tall T waves

Regression

Related to pathology

CONDITIONS IN WHICH LARGE POSITIVE T WAVES ARE FOUND

1. Posterior myocardial infarction: the high peaked T waves seen in the precordial leads are the sum of the normal upright T waves in these leads and the negative T waves—inverted—that would be recorded by an esophageal lead—i.e., the sum of the positive T wave + the mirror image of the negative posterior wall T waves.

2. Acute anterior myocardial infarction: high peaked T waves occasionally appear very early—only minutes to hours after acute anterior myocardial infarction

3. Frequent anginal attacks

4. Severe aortic stenosis

5. Left ventricular hypertrophy (LVH): high T waves occasionally appear in V_2 or V_3 when the pattern of LVH is present

6. Left bundle branch block: giant positive T waves may be seen in right precordial leads

7. Potassium intoxication: precordial T waves may become high and peaked (and duration of Q-T shortened) even before the serum level of potassium is increased

In Figure 2-18 are shown some examples of normal and of abnormal T waves, with indication of related pathology.

The U Wave

The U wave is the after potential of the T wave. It occurs at about the "super normal phase." It is at this point that ventricular premature contractions occur frequently.

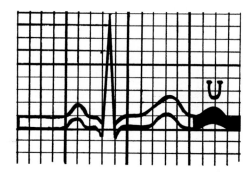

FIG. 2-19. The U wave.

The U wave begins at the end of the T wave. It follows the T wave by 0.02 to 0.04 seconds. In standard limb leads, its height is between 1 and 1.5 mm. and the duration is about 0.24 seconds. In precordial leads the amplitude, especially in V_3 or V_4, may be as high as 2.0 mm.

The polarity of the U wave is the same as the polarity of the T wave.

Prominent U waves are associated with:

Potassium deficiency

Hypercalcemia

Thyrotoxicosis

Bradycardia

Exercise

Drug effects (Digitalis; Quinidine; Epinephrine)

Negative U waves are associated with:

Infarction

Coronary insufficiency

Hypertension (23%)*

Left ventricular hypertrophy

The U wave is the repolarization of the Purkinje fibers and is considered as the T wave of the Purkinje action potential. The U wave can be separated from the T wave by carotid sinus pressure.

* Garcia-Palmieri, M. R., et al.: The significance of giant negative T waves in coronary artery disease. Am. Heart J., 52:521, 1956.

† Freundlich, J.: The diagnostic significance of tall upright T waves in the chest leads. Am. Heart J., 52:749, 1956.

* Kemp, R. L., et al.: Prognostic significance of negative U waves in the electrocardiogram in hypertension. Circulation, 15:98, 1957.

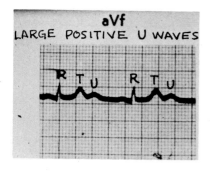

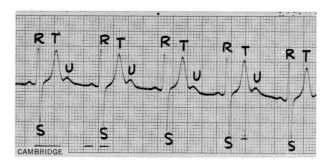

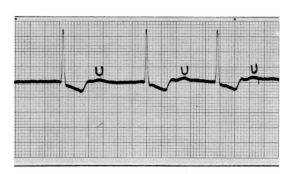

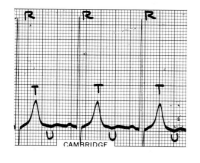

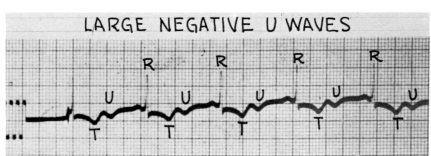

FIG. 2-20. Large positive U waves. (*Top, center*) Large U waves merging with T waves. (*Bottom*) Prominent U waves in digitalis effect.

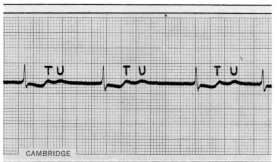

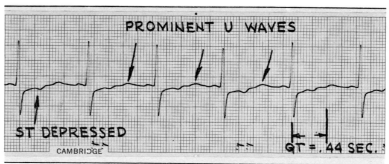

FIG. 2-21. Large negative U waves. (*Top, left*) The U waves, which follow the T wave are negative and, therefore, abnormal. The R wave is abnormally tall (amplitude 38 mm.). The T waves are peaked, pointed and symmetrical. This pattern is usually found with hypertrophy and ischemia. The negative U wave, which is a characteristic of this pattern, is always abnormal. (*Bottom*) Negative U waves in severe ischemia—coronary disease.

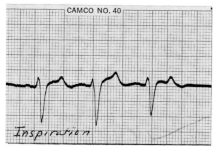

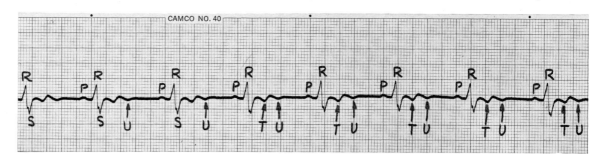

17

	P Wave Amplitude	P Wave Width	P-R Interval	Q Wave (Q% of R) Width	Q Wave (Q% of R) Depth	QRS Interval	R Wave Amplitude	S-T Segment	T Wave	U Wave Amplitude	U Wave Width
	Maximum	Maximum	0.12-0.20 sec.	Width	Depth	0.10 sec.	Maximum to Minimum	1 mm.	1-5 mm.	1.5 mm.	0.24 sec.
	2.5 mm.	0.10 sec.		Less Than 0.04 sec.	Q/R Ratio		5-16 mm.	Above or Below			
L₁					15% of R wave			1 mm. Elevation			
L₂					20% of R wave						
L₃				Up to 0.08 sec.	25% of R wave						
aVR				Up to 0.08 sec.			Less than + 4 mm.		except in this lead (T is neg.)		
aVL				Less than 0.04 sec.	25% of R wave		5-13 mm. Transverse Heart				
aVF							5-21 mm. Vertical Heart				
V₁				Up to 0.08 sec.			5-27 mm.		13 mm.		
V₂											
V₃				Less than 0.04 sec.							
V₄											
V₅											
V₆											

(S-T Segment column annotations, spanning leads: "1 mm. Elevation" (aVL–aVF region); "1-2 mm. Depression" and "2 mm. to 4 mm. Elevation" (V₁–V₅ region))

* For practical purposes, these are the upper and lower limits of the normal ECG. However, there are "gray zones" and variation from these limits may not necessarily imply abnormality.

The Q-T Interval

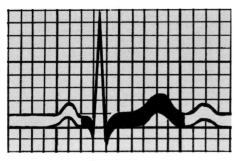

FIGURE 2-22

The Q-T interval is measured from the onset of the Q wave to the end of the T wave. It is an important feature of the electrocardiogram. Its duration has diagnostic significance: a prolonged Q-T interval indicates heart disease, just as does a prolonged P-R interval. Thus accurate measurement is important in both.

The Q-T interval is the summation of ventricular depolarization and repolarization and represents electrical systole.[1] Its duration corresponds almost exactly to the ventricular ejection time.

The Q-T interval is related to
cardiac rate
age
sex

The Q-T interval may be corrected for cardiac rate. The corrected interval (Q-T$_c$) is obtained by dividing the actual Q-T interval by the square root of the duration of one cycle (usually measured from the peak of one R wave to the peak of the next R wave):

$$Q\text{-}T_c = \frac{\text{actual Q-T interval}}{\sqrt{\text{R–R interval}}}$$

Prolonged Q-T interval may be caused by:
Prolonged overloading of the left ventricle[2]

Hypocalcemia of various etiology, including hypoparathyroidism[3]
Uremia[3]
Myocardial infarction
Quinidine[5]
Diabetic coma
Hypothermia
Hypokalemia
Hypertensive heart disease
Rheumatic heart disease
Arteriosclerotic heart disease
Coronary artery disease
Shortened Q-T interval may be caused by:
Digitalis[6]
Epinephrine
Hypercalcemia, which may be caused by
Hyperparathyroidism
Hyperkalemia

TABLE 2-3. THE Q-T INTERVAL AND THE HEART RATE*

HEART RATE (per min.)	Q-T INTERVAL (normal range) (sec.)
40–50	0.41–0.45
51–60	0.39–0.41
61–70	0.36–0.38
71–80	0.34–0.36
81–90	0.32–0.33
91–100	0.31–0.33
101–120	0.28–0.31
121–140	0.27–0.28
141–160	0.23–0.25

* After Ashman and Hull: Essentials of Electrocardiography. New York, Macmillan, 1937.

[1] Nomenclature and Criteria for Diagnosis of Diseases of the Heart. Ed. 4 p. 140. New York Heart Association, 1940.
[2] Hurst, J. W., and Wenger, N. K. (eds.): Electrocardiographic Interpretation. New York, McGraw-Hill, 1963.
[3] Bechtel, J. I., White, J. E., and Estes, E. H., Jr.: Circulation, 13:837, 1956.

Determination of Cardiac Rate

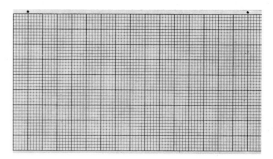

FIGURE 2-23

Cardiac rate can be determined from the electrocardiogram. On the cardiographic paper, the vertical lines, which are spaced 0.1 cm., or 1 mm. apart, are marked off at 0.04 second intervals. Every fifth line is marked more heavily, and the interval between the heavy lines is 0.5 cm. or 0.2 second. In the top margin of the paper, a heavy dot appears above every fifteenth of the heavy vertical lines, or 3 seconds apart.

These features can be used in the determination of the heart rate in the following ways:

1. Since one small square is 0.04 second wide, the number of small squares equaling 1 minute is 0.04)‾60‾, or 1,500.

Therefore the number of small squares in one R–R interval divided into 1,500 will give the heart rate per min.

(The R–R interval is measured from the peak of one R wave to the peak of the succeeding R wave.)

[4] Gunton, R. W., Scott, J. W., Lougheed, W. M., and Botterell, E. H.: Am. Heart J., 52:419, 1956.
[5] Ernstene, E. C., and Proudfit, W. L.: Am. Heart J., 38:260, 1949.
[6] Goldberger, E.: Unipolar Lead Electrocardiography and Vectorcardiography. Ed. 3. p. 164. Philadelphia, Lea & Febiger, 1953.

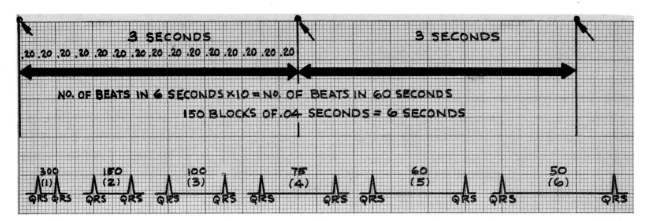

FIGURE 2-24

(1) The R-R interval is 1 large square: $\frac{300}{1} = 300$ —heart rate per min.

(2) The R-R interval is 2 large squares: $\frac{300}{2} = 150$

(3) The R-R interval is 3 large squares: $\frac{300}{3} = 100$

(4) The R-R interval is 4 large squares: $\frac{300}{4} = 75$

(5) The R-R interval is 5 large squares: $\frac{300}{5} = 60$

(6) The R-R interval is 6 large squares: $\frac{300}{6} = 50$

Should the R-R interval fall short of a square, interpolation is necessary.
For example, the R-R interval is 2½ squares:
Since R-R of 2 squares gives a rate of 150 and
R-R of 3 squares gives a rate of 100,
The difference is 50; ½ of 50 is 25; 150 minus 25 is 125
The heart rate if R-R is 2½ squares is 125 per min.

2. If a large square is 0.04 × 5, or 0.2 sec. wide, the number of large squares equaling one minute is 0.2‾)60, or 300.

Therefore the number of large squares in one R–R interval divided into 300 gives the heart rate per minute.

3. The interval between 2 dots is 15 large squares. Since 15 × 0.2 sec. is 3 seconds, the sum of two such intervals—the interval between the first dot and the third dot—is 6 seconds.

Therefore the number of complete cardiac cycles between dots 1 and 3, multiplied by 10, gives the heart rate per minute.

The number of cardiac cycles may be obtained by counting the number of P waves or R waves in the interval.

This method is very useful in the determination of ventricular or auricular rates when they are very irregular.

Applications

Regular Sinus Rhythm

Assume that the R–R interval is 3 large squares and 2 small squares, which equals 3.4 large squares.

Then 300 divided by 3.4 equals the heart rate per minute.

$$
\begin{array}{r}
88 \\
3.4\overline{)300.0} \\
272 \\
\hline
280 \\
272 \\
\end{array}
$$

or calculated by small squares:

Three large squares plus 2 small squares equals 17 small squares; 1,500 divided by 17 equals the heart rate per minute.

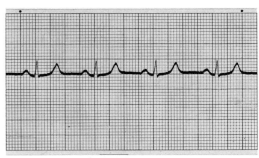

Fig. 2-25. The R-R interval measures slightly more than 4 large squares and slightly less than 21 small squares. Therefore the results obtained will not be identical.

Large squares: $4\overline{)300} = 75$ = rate per minute
$\underline{71}$
Small squares: $21\overline{)1500}$ 71 = rate per minute
$\underline{147}$
30
21

The interval measured by 3 consecutive dots is 15 cm. and represents 6 seconds. To obtain ventricular and auricular rates, multiply the number of R waves and of P waves respectively by 10. In this example, there are 7 R waves: 7 × 10 = 70 (ventricular rate per min.); and 7 P waves: 7 × 10 = 70 (auricular rate per min.).

$$\frac{88}{17 \overline{)1500}}$$
$$\frac{136}{140}$$
$$136$$

Heart rate is 88 per minute.

This is a long method, best for the beginner although it may seem to be tedious. With experience, the rate eventually can be approximated with ease in regular sinus rhythm.

Irregular Rhythm (Sinus Arrhythmia)

Irregular rhythm can be determined by the methods demonstrated above, by proper interpolation. However, if the P or the R waves are very irregular, the following procedure is useful.

Fifteen cm. are marked off with a simple metric ruler. This equals 30 large squares, or 6 seconds. To determine the rate for the R waves or the P waves, the number of R waves or P waves in the 6-second interval is multiplied by 10.

For example:

Six R waves are counted in a 15-cm. interval.

$6 \times 10 = 60$ the ventricular rate per minute.

Ten P waves are counted in the 15-cm. interval.

$10 \times 10 = 100$ the auricular rate per minute

Figure 2-24 and 2-25 further illustrate the methods described above.

CHAPTER 3

Plotting the Electrical Axis

Five Basic Patterns

There are five basic patterns that identify the portion of the heart which a particular lead faces (Fig. 3-1):

1. A qRs pattern with a negative T wave is a "back of the heart" pattern, or posterior wall pattern.

2. A qRs pattern with an upright T wave is a left ventricular epicardial pattern.

3. The RS pattern is a transitional zone pattern. The R wave is equal in amplitude to the S wave.

4. The rS pattern is a right ventricular epicardial pattern or a right ventricular cavity pattern.

5. The QS pattern is a cavity pattern: it is the pattern of the left ventricular cavity.

Generally, any one of the five basic patterns can identify the position of the electrode in relationship to the anatomical surface of the heart. Thus, a qRs pattern or a qR pattern is almost always representative of the left ventricular surface of the heart. The rS pattern and the Rs pattern may represent the right ventricular cavity of the heart and the surface of the right ventricle respectively. The RS pattern indicates that the lead is facing the interventricular septum.

"R" represents normal or high voltage.

"r" represents a low voltage.

"S" represents a deep S wave.

"s" represents a low amplitude s wave.

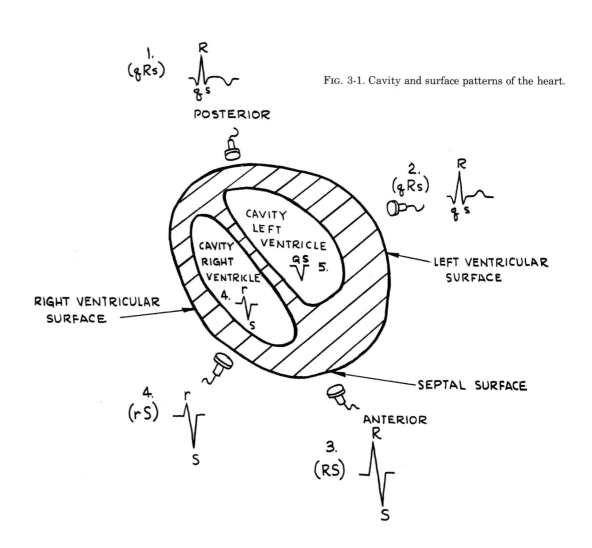

Fig. 3-1. Cavity and surface patterns of the heart.

A "Q" wave is deep in respect to the R wave.

A "q" wave is shallow in respect to the R wave.

Origin and Development of the Triaxial and the Hexaxial Systems

The three standard bipolar limb leads were introduced by Einthoven. Their polarity was fixed in such a way that the major deflection would be upright in all three leads. Thus, the leads were set up as follows:

Lead	Positive pole	Negative pole
I	left arm	right arm
II	left foot	right arm
III	left foot	left arm

Later, Einthoven proposed that the electrical field of the heart could be represented on the frontal plane of the body roughly as an equilateral triangle, with the heart—the source of the potential—at its center. Then the three standard leads could be imagined as forming the sides of the triangle (Fig. 3-2).

In Figure 3-3 the midpoint of each lead is marked, as is the center of the triangle. When the leads are superimposed at their midpoints as shown (Fig. 3-4), the triangle is "turned inside out" and the new arrangement is a triaxial system, maintaining throughout all the polarity and disposition of leads I, II and III seen in the triangle.

The unipolar limb leads have the negative terminal connected to an "indifferent" or "neutral" electrode, and the positive terminal is the "exploring" electrode (for which the lead is named). They can be represented also as a triaxial system, related to the bipolar leads as shown (Fig. 3-5). The unipolar limb lead bisects the angle formed by the two bipolar leads of which

that limb is a member, and is therefore perpendicular to the remaining bipolar lead.

The axes representing the unipolar limb leads and those representing the bipolar leads can be superimposed at their midpoint, forming a hexaxial system. All the original relationships are maintained. The angle between the pairs of bipolar leads and the angle between the pairs of unipolar

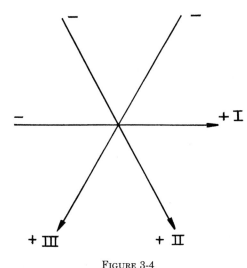

FIGURE 3-4

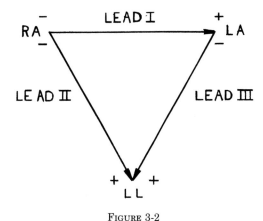

FIGURE 3-2

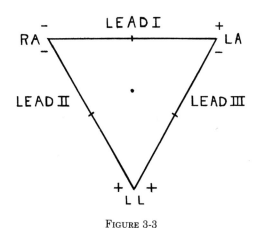

FIGURE 3-3

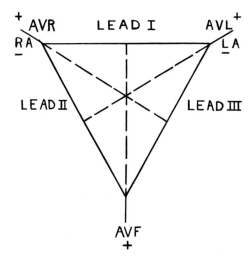

FIGURE 3-5

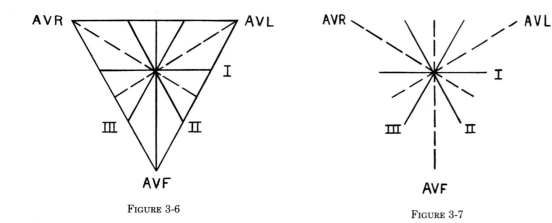

FIGURE 3-6

FIGURE 3-7

leads remain 60°. Since the unipolar leads bisect the angle formed by the bipolar leads, the adjacent angles at 0 point of the hexaxial system are all 30° (Figs. 3-6, 3-7).

Figure 3-8 shows the hexaxial system applied to a circular field. The right-hand end of lead I is taken as the zero point. From this point, readings taken clockwise are positive, those taken counterclockwise are negative. Note that in this arrangement the positive and negative designations have nothing to do with the polarity of the leads but express the mathematical relationships involved. This arrangement is very useful in the determination of the direction and magnitude of the electrical axis of the heart.

Axis Deviation

The electrical activity of the heart produces simultaneously many potentials that differ in force and direction in a three-dimensional field. The electrical potential as recorded at any given moment is the resultant—that is, the sum of the positive and the negative potentials present at that moment. Such a force, having direction as well as magnitude, is a vector. The vector that is the resultant of all the forces acting at a given moment represents the electrical axis of the heart. The QRS vector represents the resultant of forces in the ventricle. Vectors of P waves and of T waves also may be calculated from the electrocardiogram or the vectorcardiogram.

When a vector is plotted graphically on a system of coordinates, the length of the line represents the magnitude of the force and its position indicates the direction (see Fig. 3-8). In the normal heart the axis will be found to lie between 0° and 90°. A position between 0° and −90° demonstrates left axis deviation; between 90° and 180° in-

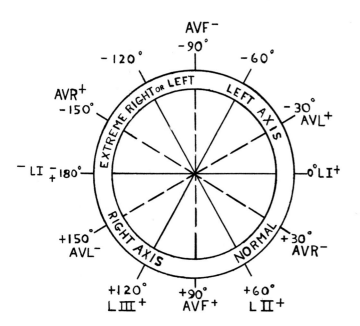

FIGURE 3-8

Normal axis   0 to 90°
Left axis   0 to −30°
Right axis   90° to 180°
Extreme right axis   180° to −90°
Extreme left axis   −90° to −180°

dicates right axis deviation. Left or right axis deviation may indicate structural abnormality or a pathologic state. In adults, left axis deviation of between −30° and −90° usually is indicative of severe myocardial pathology.

Conditions Associated with Left Axis Deviation

Elevated diaphragm (commonly associated with endomorphism)
Chronic hypertension
Chronic aortic regurgitation
Left bundle branch block
Myocardial infarction
Interventricular septal defect
Coarctation of the aorta
Mitral insufficiency

Conditions Associated with Right Axis Deviation

Vertical heart in normal persons
Mitral stenosis
Cor pulmonale, acute or chronic
Acute myocardial infarction (lateral wall infarction)
Right bundle branch block
Congenital defects
    Pulmonary stenosis
    Dextrocardia
    Ostium primum septal defect
    Ebstein's disease
    Tetralogy of Fallot

In the following section a number of procedures for the determination of axis deviation are presented. The results obtained are very close approximations of those given by more elaborate methods and will give the information important to the interpretation of the cardiogram and to diagnosis based on the data obtained from the cardiogram. Therefore the numerical value of the axis deviation (which may be expressed in degrees) should be calculated for the QRS vector of every cardiogram and recorded, so that serial changes that may be of diagnostic significance will not be overlooked.

Methods for Determining Axis Deviation

Axis Deviation by Major Deflection

Upright major deflections in both lead I and lead III indicate that axis deviation is in the normal range (Fig. 3-9 A).

Upright major deflection in lead I and inversion of the major deflection in lead III indicates generally left axis deviation (Fig. 3-9 B).

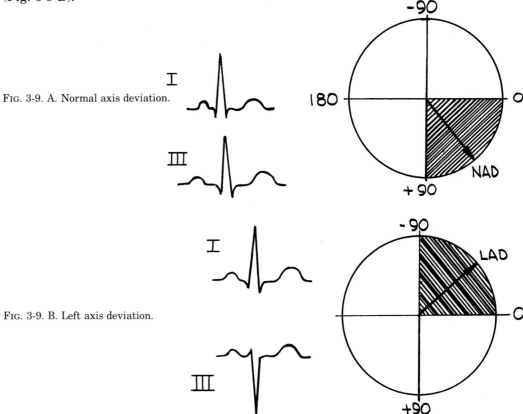

FIG. 3-9. A. Normal axis deviation.

FIG. 3-9. B. Left axis deviation.

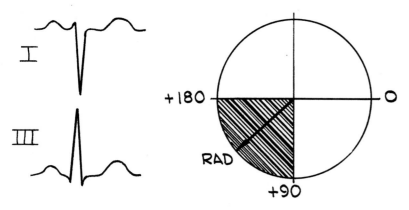

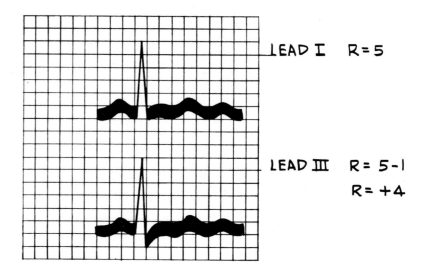

FIG. 3-9. C. Right axis deviation.

Inversion of the major deflection in lead I, with upright major deflection in lead III indicates roughly right axis deviation (Fig. 3-9 C).

Since this method is only a general indicator and is not always reliable, other methods are used to locate the electrical axis more precisely.

Plotting the Value of the Major Deflection in Lead I and Lead III

Measure the amplitude of R and of S in lead I and in lead III.

Add the values of R and S in lead I.

Using the Bayley triaxial system, mark off from the zero point on lead I the point representing the net value obtained, and repeat the procedure for the sum of R and S in lead III.

Drop perpendiculars from these two points.

Draw an arrow from the zero point to the point of intersection of the perpendiculars. This arrow represents the QRS axis.

Axis deviation is measured by the angle between 0° and the QRS axis.

This procedure is illustrated in Figures 3-10, 3-11 and 3-12.

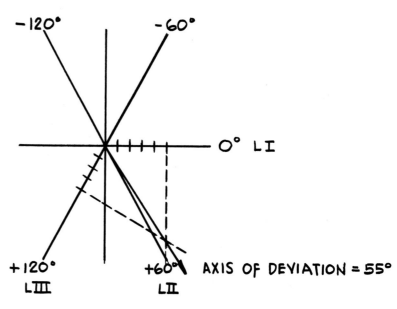

FIG. 3-10. Normal axis deviation.

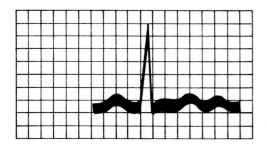

LEAD I R = 6

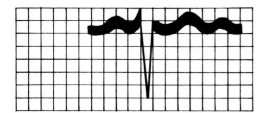

LEAD III R = -5 + 1
R = -4

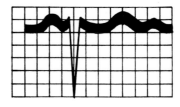

LEAD I R = -5 + 1
R = -4

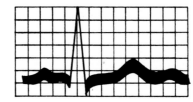

LEAD III R = 5 - 1
R = +4

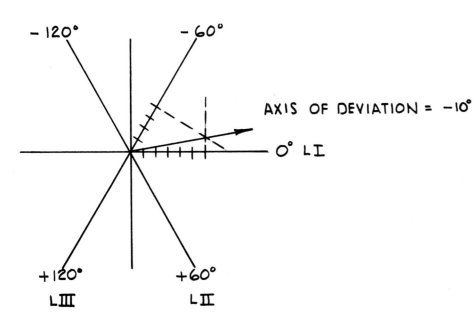

Fig. 3-11. Left axis deviation.

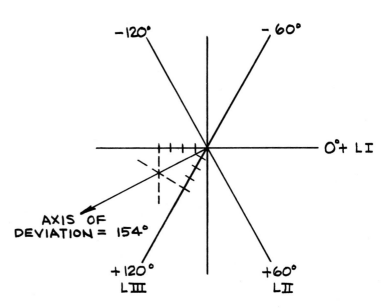

Fig. 3-12. Right axis deviation.

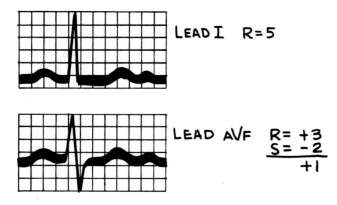

LEAD I   R=5

LEAD AVF   R= +3
S= -2
—
+1

FIGURE 3-13

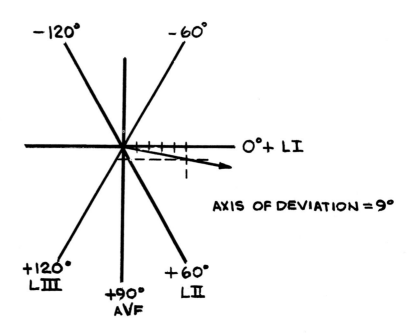

AXIS OF DEVIATION = 9°

Plotting the Major Deflections in Lead I and aVF (Fig. 3-13)

Using the hexaxial system, the value of R plus s in lead I and of R plus s in aVF are plotted on the appropriate axis. Perpendiculars are dropped from these points. An arrow drawn from zero point to the point of intersection of the perpendiculars will indicate QRS axis deviation.

Using the rs Pattern (Fig. 3-14)

A vector force will produce the greatest deflection in the lead which is most nearly parallel to it. It will produce a zero net deflection (an equiphasic, or rs, pattern) in the lead to which the force is perpendicular. (See Fig. 3-14)

The hexaxial system clearly depicts the vector relationships of the extremity leads (see Fig. 3-6). The pairs of perpendiculars can be seen to be lead I and aVF; lead II and aVL; and lead III and aVR (Fig. 3-7). An rs pattern in one member of a pair indicates that the electrical axis is directed along the other member. Therefore, in an electrocardiogram that shows an rs pattern

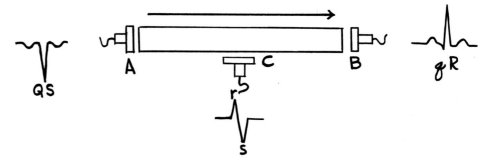

FIGURE 3-14

in a limb lead, the lead perpendicular to the one in which the rs pattern appears can be taken as the electrical axis. For example, if rs is found in lead I, the electrical axis is parallel to aVF. The net value (plus or minus) of the major deflection in aVF determines the direction of the electrical axis, which would be 90° or −90°, accordingly. (See Fig. 3-8)

This method is accurate only for patterns that show rs in standard and unipolar limb leads. When no (rs) pattern is present, one of the methods presented previously should be used.

CHAPTER 4

Sinus Rhythms, Sinus Arrhythmias, and Atrial Rhythms

Sinus Rhythm and Sinus Arrhythmias

The normal heart has two types of rhythm:
(1) regular sinus rhythm
(2) irregular sinus rhythm
Irregular sinus rhythm is called Sinus Arrhythmia. The cardiac respiratory center influences respiration. Inspiration and expiration cause variation of regular and irregular sinus rhythms.

The normal heart rate varies with age. In adults it is between 72 and 80, in young children 100, and after 60 years of age it may be as high as 100 beats per minute.

Sinus Rhythm

Sinus Rhythm at Various Rates

1. 36-60 — Sinus Bradycardia
2. 60-100 — Sinus Normocardia
3. 100-150 — Sinus Tachycardia

A rise of 1°F. in temperature causes a rise of 10 beats per minute in the cardiac rate.

Regular Sinus Rhythm, ECG Criteria

1. Sinus rhythm must originate in the sino-auricular node (P-R relationship must be normal—i.e., a p wave must be followed by a QRS at regular intervals).
2. The P wave must be normal.
3. The QRS interval must be normal.

In regular sinus rhythm, the P–P interval or the R–R interval establishes a specific interval which should not vary more than 0.16 second. If the variation is 0.16 sec. or greater, then a sinus arrhythmia is present. The R–R interval is known as the sphygmic interval or the intersystolic interval.

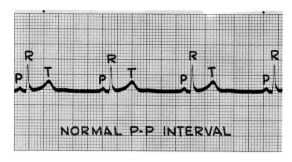

FIG. 4-2. The normal sinus rhythm electrocardiogram.

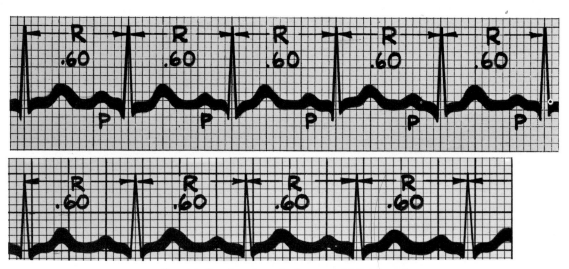

FIG. 4-1. Regular sinus rhythm: equal P-P intervals and equal R-R intervals and regular P-QRS sequence.

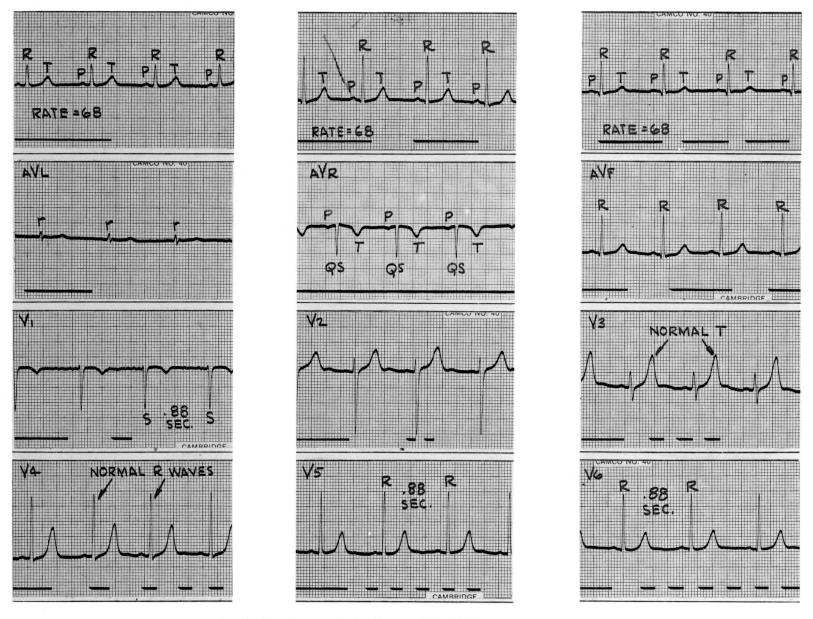

Fɪɢ. 4-3. Regular sinus rhythm. Note regular P–QRS relationship in all leads.

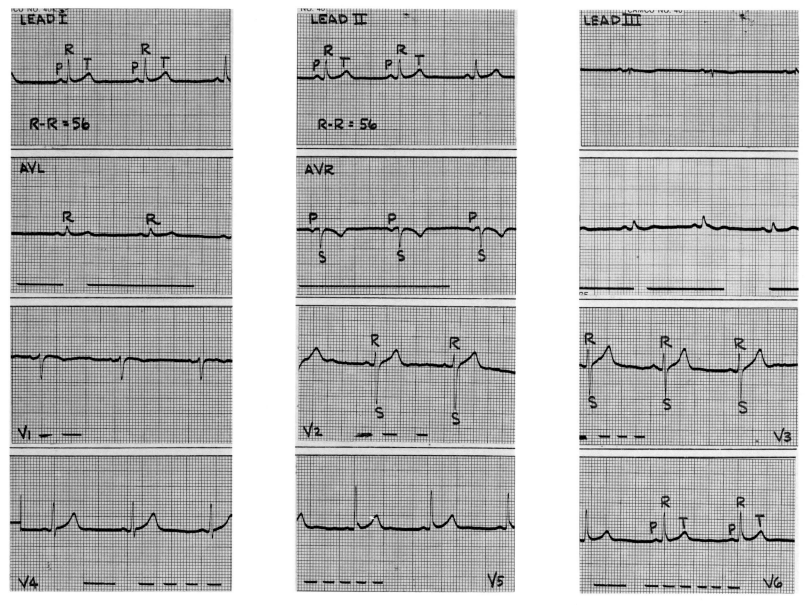

FIGURE 4-4

FIGS. 4-3 and 4-4. Examples of normal regular sinus rhythm (sinus normocardia). Note regular P-QRS relationship in all leads. 56 = rate/min.

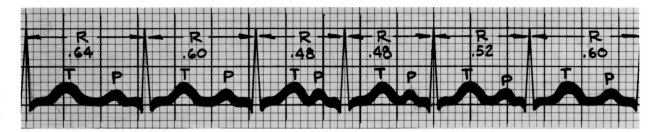

FIGURE 4-5
Sinus Arrhythmia

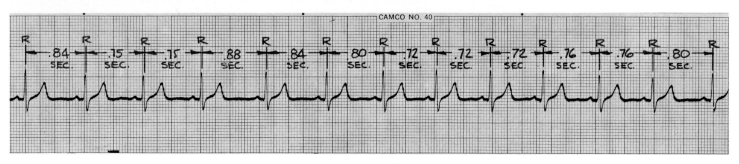

Sinus Arrhythmia

Definition

Sinus arrhythmia is a slightly irregular rhythm originating in the sino-auricular node. It varies periodically with respiration: the heart rate increases with inspiration and decreases with expiration.

FIG. 4-6. Sinus arrhythmia.
  Shortest R-R — 0.72 sec. (18 × 0.04).
  Longest R-R — 0.88 sec. (22 × 0.04)
  Difference — 0.16 sec.
  Variation in R-R interval of 0.16 sec. or more is considered sinus arrhythmia.

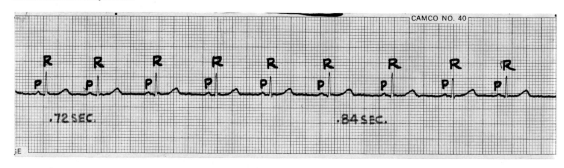

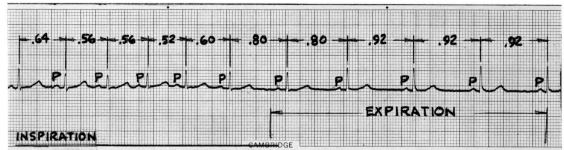

FIG. 4-7. (Above) P-P interval varies, but only by 0.12 second. (Left) R-R interval varies, from 0.92 sec. (maximum) to 0.52 sec. (minimum). Note that variation corresponds to phase of respiration.

Criteria

P–P interval or R–R interval varies in
duration by at least 0.16 sec.

Heart rate—40 to 100 beats per min.

It tends to appear at slower rates and dis-
appear at higher rates.

Associated with:

Active rheumatic fever

Infectious diseases

Atelectasis

Chronic adhesive pleuritis

Intracranial tension

Digitalization

Normal in children and young adults

Figures 4-7 to 4-9 give examples of sinus
arrhythmia.

Differentiate sinus arrhythmia from normal sinus rhythm (Figs. 4-7, A and B),
using the criteria given above.

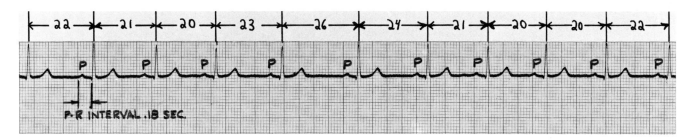

Fig. 4-8. A. The R-R interval is wide, and the difference between the longest and the shortest
R-R interval shown is 0.24 sec.

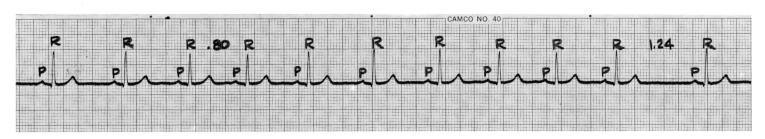

Fig. 4-8. B. Shortest R-R interval —0.80 sec.; longest R-R interval —1.24 sec. Difference —0.44
sec., indicating sinus arrhythmia.

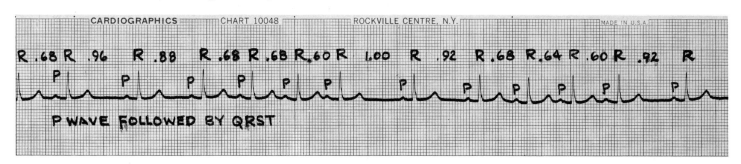

Fig. 4-9. Marked sinus arrhythmia. Note periodic recurrence of long and of short cycles. R-R
interval varies from a minimum of 0.60 sec. to a maximum of 1.00 sec.

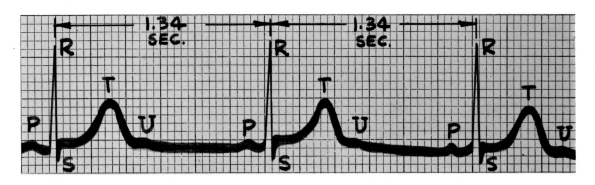

FIG. 4-10. Sinus bradycardia.

Sinus Bradycardia

Sinus bradycardia is a regular sinus rhythm originating in the sino-auricular node. The rate is slowed as a result of vagal stimulation of the cardiac regulatory center via the decelerator fibers so that the rate is 60, or less, per minute.

Physiologic Bradycardia

Found in
  Laborers and trained athletes
  Emotional states leading to syncope

Carotid sinus pressure; eyeball pressure; intracranial pressure
Sleep

Sinus Bradycardia May Also Be Associated with

Systemic disease
  Obstructive jaundice
  Obstructive diseases of the intestine, kidney or bladder

During convalescence after some diseases marked by fever (e.g., influenza)
Myxedema
Cardiac arrest: *it is the earliest warning in 80 per cent of cardiac arrests during surgery*
Myocardial infarction (may be an early clue)
Drug action
  Digitalis
  Morphine
  Quinidine
  Anesthesia

FIG. 4-11. A. The area measured by three consecutive dots (30 large squares) contains 5 complete cardiac cycles (R-R interval): therefore the heart rate is 5 × 10, or 50—sinus bradycardia. R-R interval is constant—regular sinus rhythm. P-R relationship (interval) is constant.

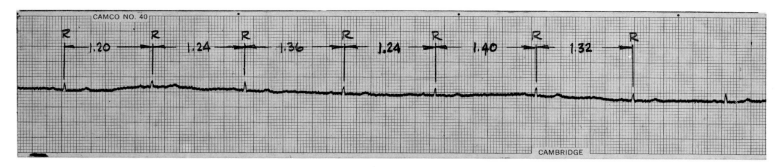

FIG. 4-11. B. R-R interval is 1.20 sec. or more: heart rate of less than 50 per min. P-R relationship is normal. T waves are flattened. Q-T interval is of normal duration. Note sinus arrhythmia.

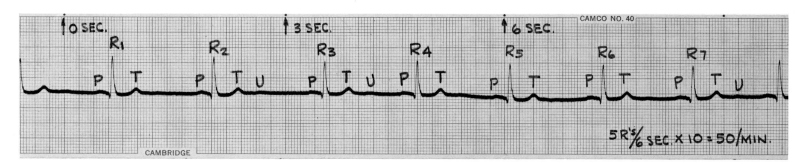

FIG. 4-12. (A) Sinus bradycardia with sinus arrhythmia.

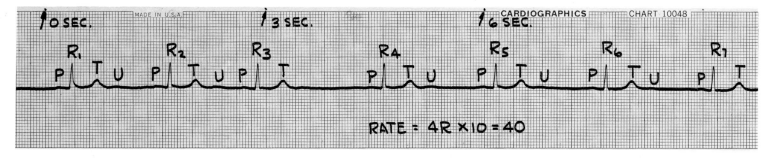

FIG. 4-12. (B) Rate of P wave (or R wave) is less than 60, therefore this is a sinus bradycardia. Note normal P-R relationship.

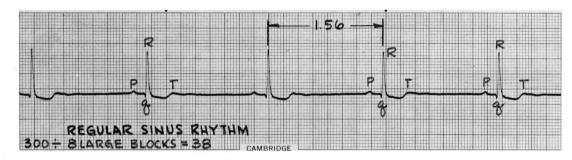

FIG. 4-13 A. Sinus bradycardia with regular sinus rhythm. A. R-R is 1.56 sec. and regular. Rate of heart beat is 38 (ventricular rate and auricular rate).

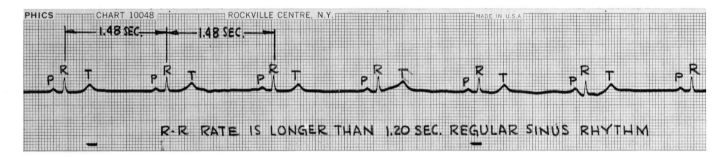

FIG. 4-13 B. The sinus bradycardia is associated with a chronic myocardial infarction. R-R is 1.48 sec. and regular. Heart rate is 40.

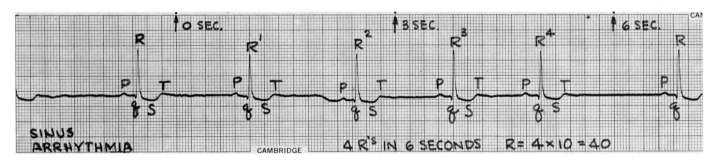

FIG. 4-13 C. Sinus bradycardia with sinus arrhythmia. Rate may be calculated by counting the number of QRS complexes in a 6-second interval.

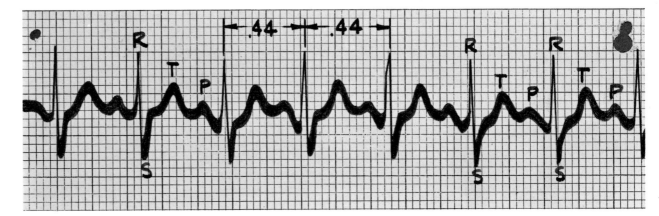

FIG. 4-14. Sinus tachycardia.

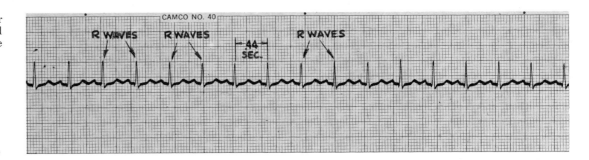

FIG. 4-15. Sinus tachycardia, with a rate of 140 per minute. All R waves are equidistant, the R-R interval being 0.44 sec. P-P interval is 0.44 sec. Cycles are normal.

Electrocardiographic Criteria (see Figs. 4-11–4-13)

Heart rate – 60, or less, per minute
   (R–R interval or P–P interval is 1.0 sec.
   or more, measuring over 5 large squares;
   rate of P waves and of R waves is 60
   per min. or less)
P-R relationship – normal
T waves may be flattened
Q-T interval is longer than usual
U wave may be prominent

Sinus Tachycardia

Sinus tachycardia is a regular sinus rhythm, with a rate of at least 100 per minute and rarely exceeding 160 per minute.

Factors Associated with Sinus Tachycardia

Physiologic
   Exercise

Strong emotion
Pain
Anxiety states
Pathologic
   Fever
   Hyperthyroidism
   Hemorrhage
   Shock
   Anemia
   Infection
   Congestive heart failure
Other factors
   Drugs
      Epinephrine (sympathomimetic drug)
      Atropine
      Meperidine (I.V.)

Food, etc.
   Tea
   Coffee
   Alcohol
   Tobacco

Electrocardiographic Criteria

P-R relationship is constant.
Rhythm is a regular sinus rhythm.
The atrial and the ventricular rates are between 100 and 160.
The R–R interval (or the P–P interval) is 0.60 second or less in duration. (On the ECG, 3 large squares or less: 3×0.20 sec. = 0.60 sec.)

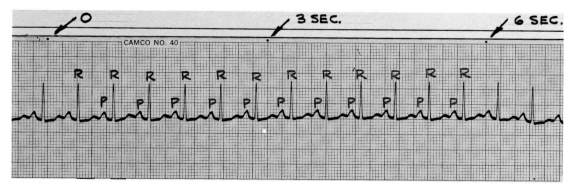

Fɪɢ. 4-16. (*Left*). The tracing shows normal sinus P waves; equal P-P intervals; and 12 R waves in 6-second intervals 10 × 12 = 120: sinus tachycardia, with a rate of 120 beats per min.

Fɪɢ. 4-17. (*Below*). ECG fulfilling criteria of sinus tachycardia:

T-P interval is short. P waves, R waves and T waves are normal. P-R relationship is normal. Therefore, sinus mechanism is operative (i.e., impulses have their origin in the sino-auricular node and the sequence of conduction is normal). R-R intervals are equal and less than 0.6 sec. in duration. There are 12 R waves in the strip measured between the first and the third dot. The rate is 12 × 10, or 120 beats per min., and the rhythm is therefore a sinus tachycardia.

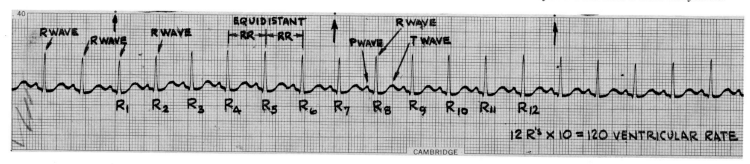

50 — The "Magic Number"

In regard to rate, all cardiac rhythms may be classified roughly by multiples of 50 (see table at right). Although there are overlapping zones, for practical purposes this method is helpful.

The More Common Atrial Arrhythmias

The atria are composed of cardiac muscle and have all the physiological functions and activities characteristic of cardiac tissue. The most common disturbances of the atria

occur in the muscle and may be the result of disease processes.

The most common disturbances of atrial rhythm are:

    Atrial premature systoles
    Atrial tachycardia
    Atrial flutter
    Atrial fibrillation

In itself, each ectopic rhythm may be innocent or innocuous. However, if there is underlying pathology, one arrhythmia may herald the development of another and more serious arrhythmia. Hypothetically, a series

TABLE 4-1. CLASSIFICATIONS OF CARDIAC RHYTHMS BY MULTIPLES OF 50

HEART RATE	CARDIAC RHYTHM	
0–50	sinus bradycardia	idioventricular rhythm AV nodal rhythm
50–100	normocardia (sinus rhythm)	
100–150	sinus tachycardia	nodal tachycardia
150–250	atrial tachycardia	ventricular tachycardia
250–350	atrial flutter	
350–600	atrial fibrillation	

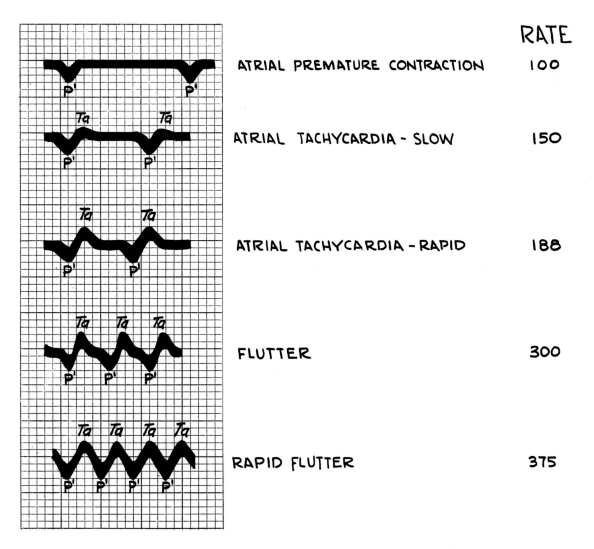

	RATE
ATRIAL PREMATURE CONTRACTION	100
ATRIAL TACHYCARDIA - SLOW	150
ATRIAL TACHYCARDIA - RAPID	188
FLUTTER	300
RAPID FLUTTER	375

INVERTED P WAVES BECOMING F WAVES
ISOELECTRIC LINE DISAPPEARS IN FLUTTER

Fig. 4-18. Analysis of flutter wave. Note inverted P waves becoming F waves. Isoelectric line disappears in flutter.

of pathologic events might result in the following course:

Atrial premature systoles may increase in rate and number, or one or two premature atrial contractions may be followed immediately by a paroxysm of atrial tachycardia, which continues at a higher rate (150–250). If the rate increases still more (250–350), the result is atrial flutter. The atrial flutter may become more advanced and chaotic and convert to atrial fibrillation with a rate that is irregular and very high (350–600).

Atrial Extrasystoles

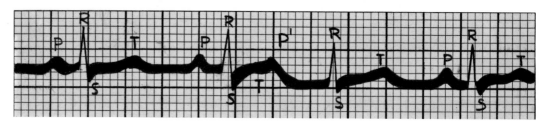

FIG. 4-19. P' indicates atrial extrasystole.

Synonyms: Premature atrial systoles. Premature atrial contractions.

Definition: Atrial extrasystoles are atrial contractions that are premature, occurring as a result of stimuli that originate in the atria rather than in the sino-auricular node. That is, the focus of origin is an ectopic, abnormal focus.

Factors Associated with Atrial Extrasystoles

Pathologic
    Rheumatic heart disease (may be fore-runner to atrial fibrillation)
    Pulmonary heart disease
    Pulmonary disease (with hypoxia): bronchitis; bronchiectasis; asthma; lung abscess
    Myocardial infarction
    Arteriosclerotic heart disease
Drug actions
    General anesthesia
    Digitalis
    Epinephrine
    Diuretics (causing hypokalemia)
Food, etc.
    Tea; coffee; alcohol; tobacco
    Psychic stress; emotion; fatigue

The ECG Findings

1. The P wave appears prematurely.
2. The premature P wave differs in contour from the normal P wave in the same lead.
3. The P-R interval may be prolonged.
4. The P' wave may be inverted.

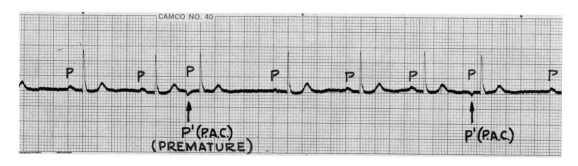

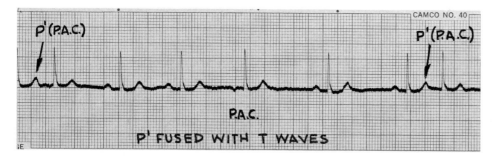

FIG. 4-20. (*Top* and *Bottom*) Examples of ECG patterns showing atrial extrasystoles. P.A.C.— premature atrial contraction. (Premature atrial waves may also be indicated by the symbol P'.)

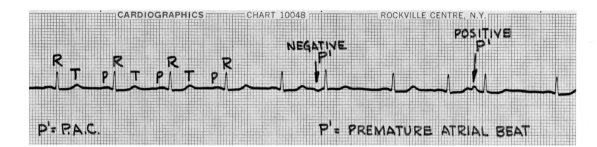

NEGATIVE P'

POSITIVE P'

P' = P.A.C.   P' = PREMATURE ATRIAL BEAT

Fig. 4-21. Premature atrial contractions. P'–premature beat. QRS resembles basic QRS. P' may be upright or negative. P-R interval is greater than 0.10 sec. P wave rhythm is interrupted.

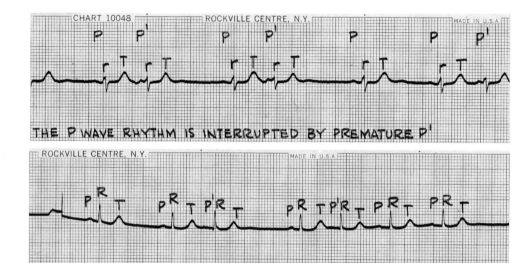

THE P WAVE RHYTHM IS INTERRUPTED BY PREMATURE P'

Fig. 4-22. Atrial premature beats in bigeminy. The P wave rhythm is interrupted by the premature P'.

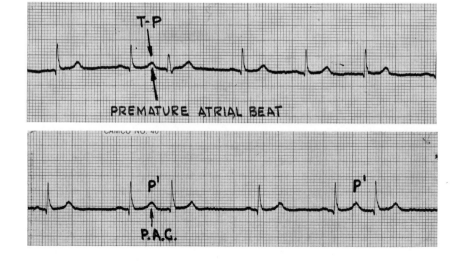

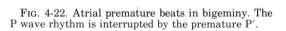

T-P

PREMATURE ATRIAL BEAT

P'

P.A.C.

Fig. 4-23. (A) Examples of premature atrial beat. T-P represents merging of T wave with premature P wave.

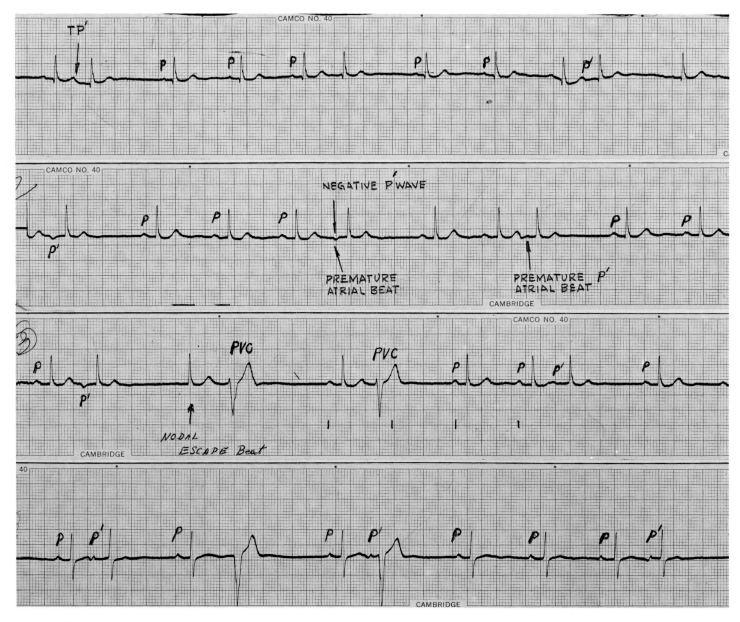

FIG. 4-23. (B) Premature atrial beats. P' represents premature atrial beats.

5. The regularity of the normal P wave rhythm is interrupted.
6. There may be some distortion of the preceding T wave by the premature P wave.
7. The ventricular complex is usually normal but may be aberrant in form if the premature atrial beat coincides with the refractory phase of any ventricular beat.
8. The sum of the interval including the preextrasystolic and the post-extra-systolic interval is less than 2 normal R–R intervals.

Atrial Tachycardia*†

Atrial tachycardia is a rapid, regular rhythm with a rate of 150-250. The impulses originating from foci in the atria away from the sino-atrial node trigger runs of premature systoles with abrupt onset and abrupt termination. The P′ is different from the dominant sinus P wave, but resembles the sino-auricular P wave in contour.

This ectopic rhythm, which is observed more frequently in office practice than in hospital practice, may last for minutes, hours, days, weeks or months.

Factors Related to Atrial Tachycardia

Emotional stress
Drug action
   Digitalis
   Quinidine
   Aspirin, etc.

* Katz, L. N., and Pick, A.: Clinical Electrocardiography. Part 1. Arrhythmias. pp. 172-175. Philadelphia, Lea and Febiger, 1956.
† Wilson, F. N.: Arch. Int. Med., 16:1008, 1915.

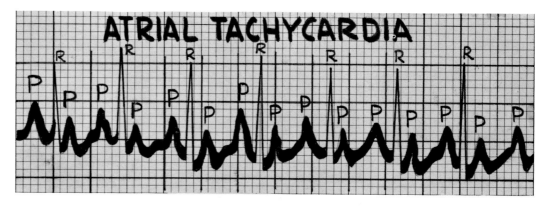

FIGURE 4-24

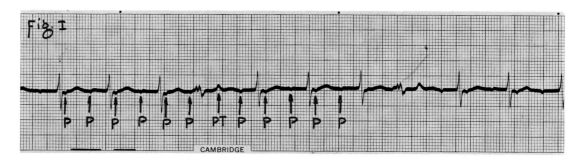

FIG. 4-25, I. Atrial Tachycardia. P wave rate is 170.

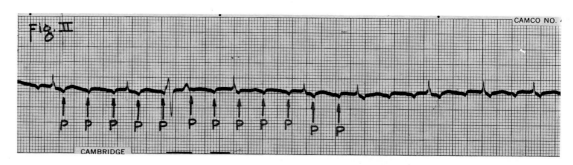

FIG. 4-25, II. Atrial tachycardia. Lead S-5 (Lewis lead). P waves are more obvious and prominent.

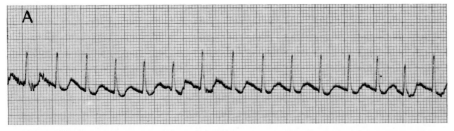

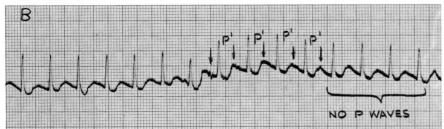

Fig. 4-26. Atrial tachycardia. A. Ventricular rate 150-160. P wave is imposed on T wave. B. Note disappearance of P wave.

Fig. 4-26. C. Rate 150. There is T-P merging. D. Cessation of tachycardia reveals P waves that are normal but slightly prolonged in duration.

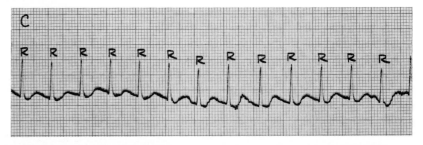

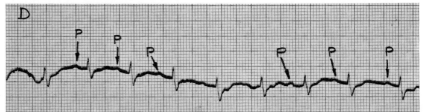

Fig. 4-27. (Below) Atrial tachycardia. T and P waves are merged. P' rate is 160. Note separation of P wave and T wave at conversion to normal sinus rhythm.

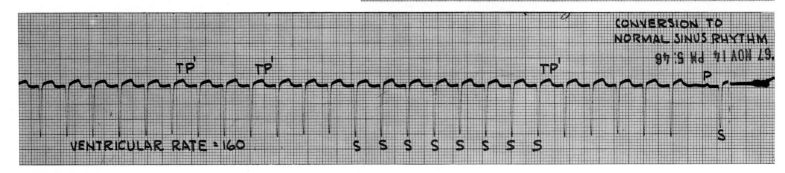

Stimulants etc.
  Tobacco
  Coffee
  Tea
  Alcohol

Cardiac disease
  Thyrotoxic heart disease
  Recent infarction
  Coronary artery disease

Rheumatic heart disease (atrial tachycardia may be forerunner of atrial fibrillation or Wolf-Parkinson-White syndrome)

ECG Criteria

P' wave rate is between 150 and 250.
P' waves do not differ much in contour from sinus P waves but are not retrograde.

P' wave may not be identifiable.

Paroxysm may be preceded by an atrial extrasystole; termination of paroxysm may be followed by an atrial extrasystole.

Since bundle branches become refractory, ventricular aberration is common.

Relationship between T waves and P waves is constant.

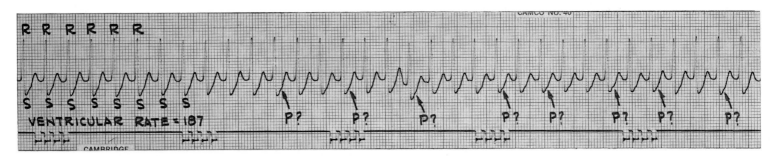

Fig. 4-28. The focus of origin of this tachycardia cannot be identified with certainty in this ECG. Therefore the arrhythmia can be classified only as supraventricular tachycardia (atrial tachycardia?).

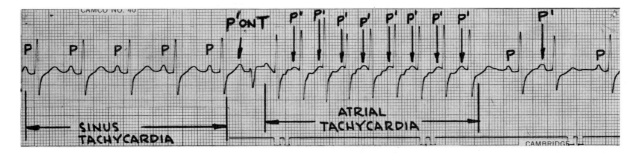

Fig. 4-29. Paroxysm of atrial tachycardia, preceded by sinus rhythm, begins abruptly and terminates as abruptly, with return to sinus rhythm. This is an unusual tracing: it is very seldom that the beginning of a paroxysm is caught on an ECG. Note P' on T wave.

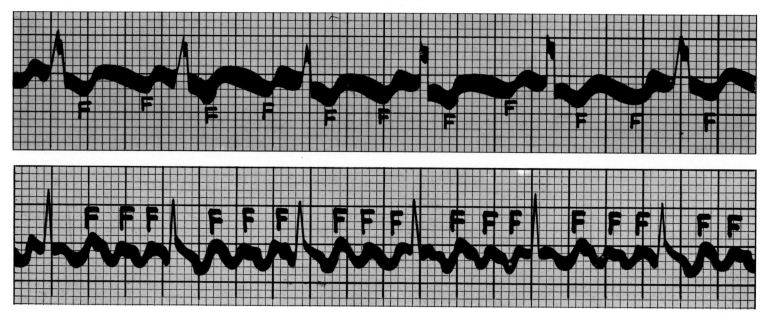

FIG. 4-30. Atrial flutter.

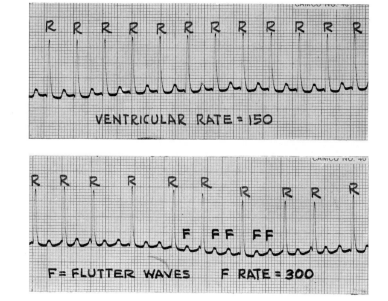

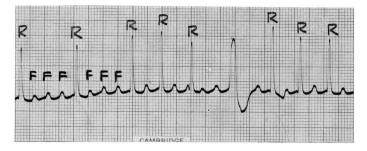

FIG. 4-31. Atrial flutter.

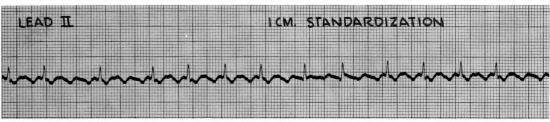

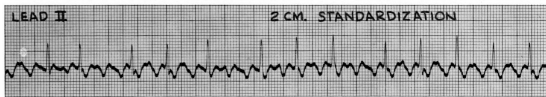

FIG. 4-32. Atrial flutter exposed by increased standardization. Note saw-tooth appearance in double standardization.

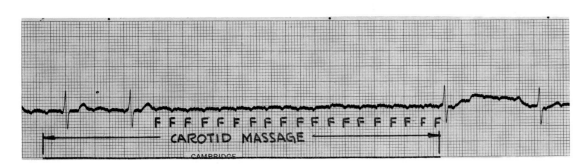

FIG. 4-33. Atrial flutter with carotid sinus massage, identified by the regularity and rate of F waves.

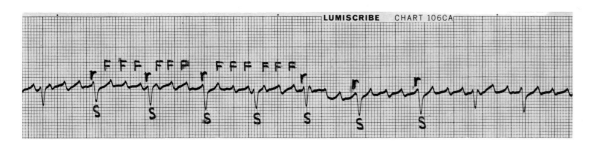

FIG. 4-34. 4:1 flutter.

Atrial Flutter*

Atrial flutter is a rapid regular atrial rhythm, arising from an excitable ectopic focus in the atria and with a rate ranging from 250 to 350. The atrial beat is regular and is inscribed as a saw-tooth or regular undulating F wave. The ventricular rate may vary and the ventricles may respond after every contraction or after every second, third or fourth atrial contraction.

Factors Associated with Atrial Flutter

Rheumatic heart disease, particularly with mitral stenosis
Coronary artery disease
Hypertensive heart disease
Arteriosclerotic heart disease
Hyperthyroidism
Pneumonia

ECG Criteria

1. Presence of saw-tooth flutter wave
2. Flutter waves seen best in leads II, III, aVF and V_1 and V_2 (continued on page 49.)

* Cecil and Loeb: Textbook of Medicine. ed. 10. p. 1306. Philadelphia, W. B. Saunders, 1959.

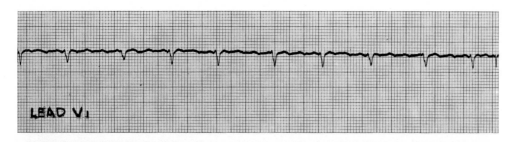

LEAD V₁

LEAD V₁   R RATE = 90
          F RATE = 300

Fɪɢ. 4-35. Atrial flutter.

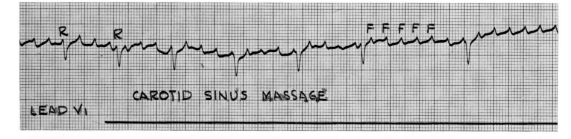

R   R   F F F F F

CAROTID SINUS MASSAGE

LEAD V₁

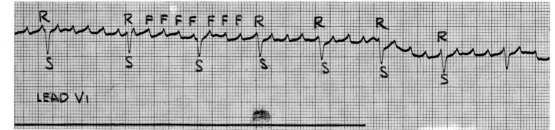

R   R F F F F F F F R   R   R
S   S   S   S   S   R
                                              S

LEAD V₁

Fɪɢ. 4-36. (*Below*) Atrial flutter.

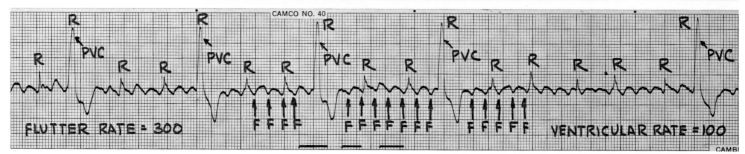

R   R   R   R   R
R   PVC   R   R   PVC   R   R   PVC   R   R   R   R   R   PVC
                              R   R   PVC
FLUTTER RATE = 300   F F F F   F F F F F F F   F F F F F   VENTRICULAR RATE = 100

CAMCO NO. 40

CAMB

48

3. Regular atrial rhythm with a rate of 250-350
4. Ventricular response of 1:1, 2:1, 3:1, 4:1 or higher
5. F waves always uniform in size, shape and frequency
6. Absence of isoelectric line

Atrial Fibrillation

Atrial fibrillation is an arrhythmia originating from one or more ectopic foci in the atria. The rate is exceedingly high (400 to 600) and the beat is totally irregular ("irregular irregularity"), creating the pattern of f (Fibrillatory) waves. The ventricular response also is irregular, with rates of 50 to 200.

Atrial fibrillation may occur in normal hearts, usually as a transient episode.

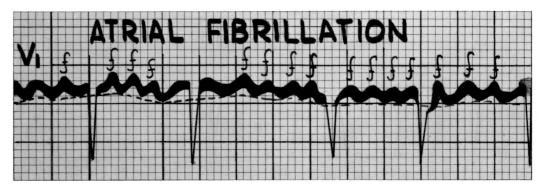

FIGURE 4-37. (*Above*)

FIG. 4-38. (*Below*) Atrial fibrillation (impure flutter).

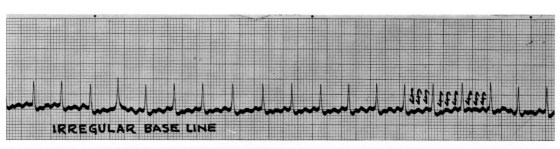

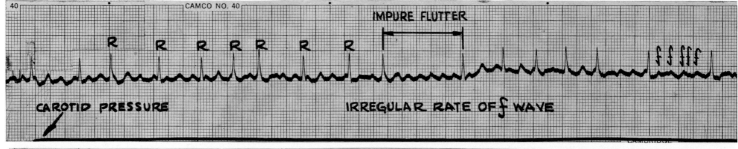

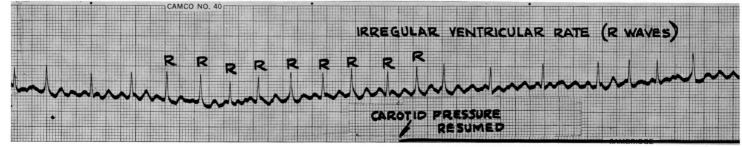

Factors Associated with Atrial Fibrillation

Commonly found in
   Hyperthyroidism (20% of cases)
   Rheumatic heart disease
   Cardiorespiratory disease
Other Cardiac Pathology
   Hypertensive heart disease
   Arteriosclerotic heart disease
   Preceding or accompanying acute myo-
     cardial infarction

   Neoplastic invasion of the atria
Miscellaneous
   Anesthesia
   Surgery
   Infection

Electrocardiographic Criteria

1. Absence of clear P waves and P-R intervals
2. P waves replaced by f waves
3. f waves:
   irregular in size, shape, and spacing
   rate between 400 and 600
   configuration variable, fine to coarse
   often difficult to impossible to discern
4. Base line — undulatory

Figures 4-38 to 4-45 should be studied for the various characteristics of fibrillation to be found in the ECG.

FIG. 4-39. (*Below*) Atrial fibrillation with rapid ventricular rate. Note absence of P waves; total irregularity of R waves. Ventricular rate — 130.

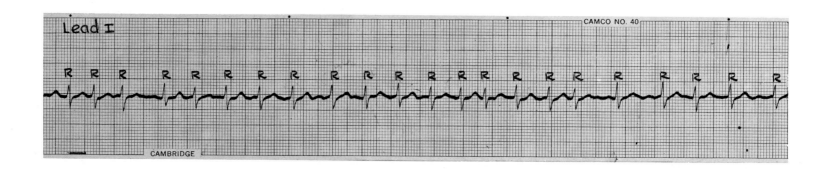

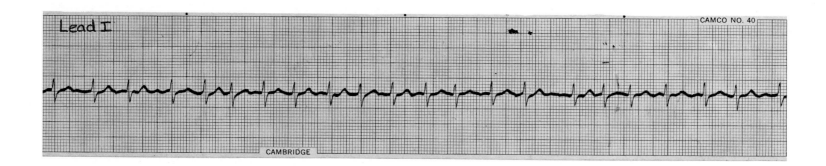

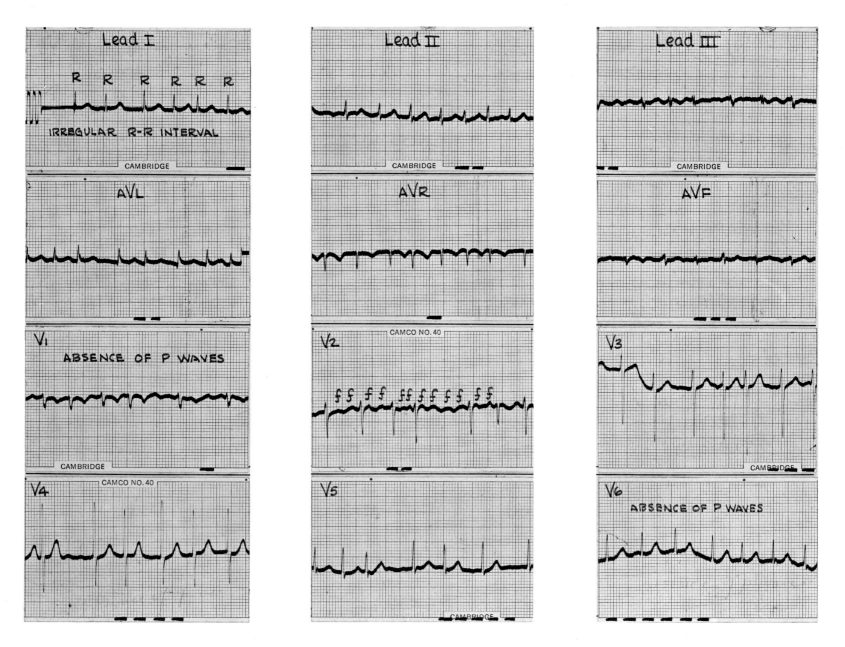

Fig. 4-40. Atrial fibrillation. Note that some characteristics are seen better in some leads than they are in others. P and P-R intervals are absent. Note irregularity of R rate.

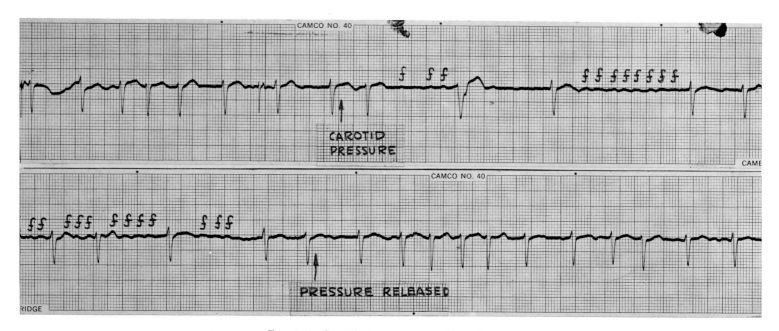

FIG. 4-41. Carotid sinus pressure widens the ventricular irregularity in V₁; f waves become more prominent.

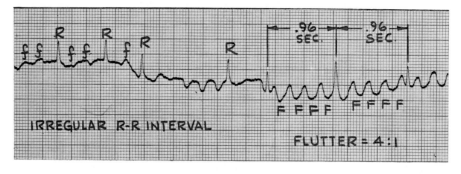

FIG. 4-42. Fibrillation — flutter.

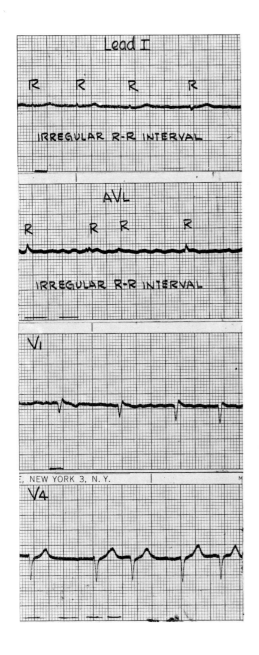

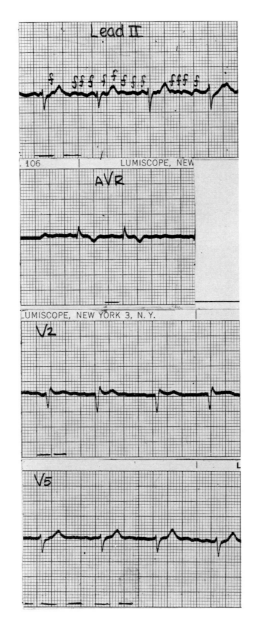

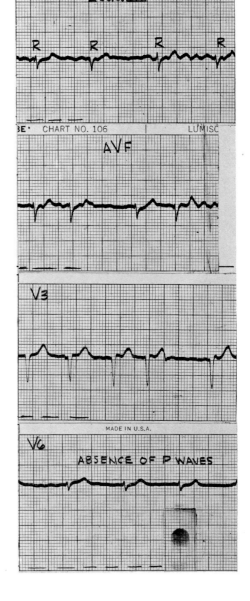

FIG. 4-43. Atrial fibrillation.

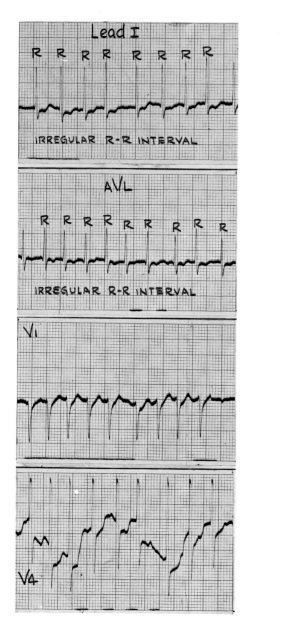

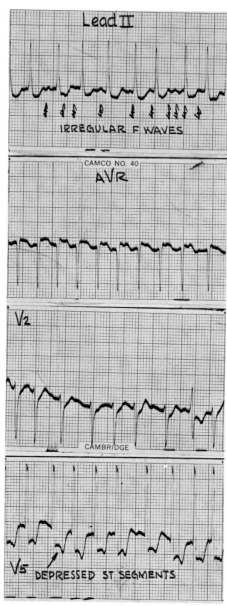

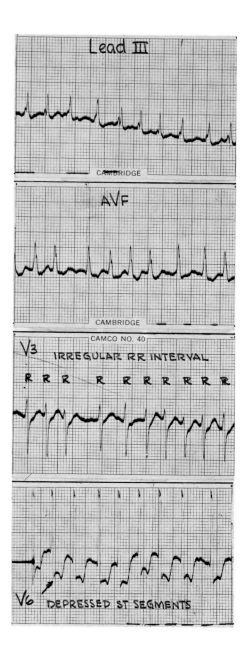

FIG. 4-44. Atrial fibrillation.

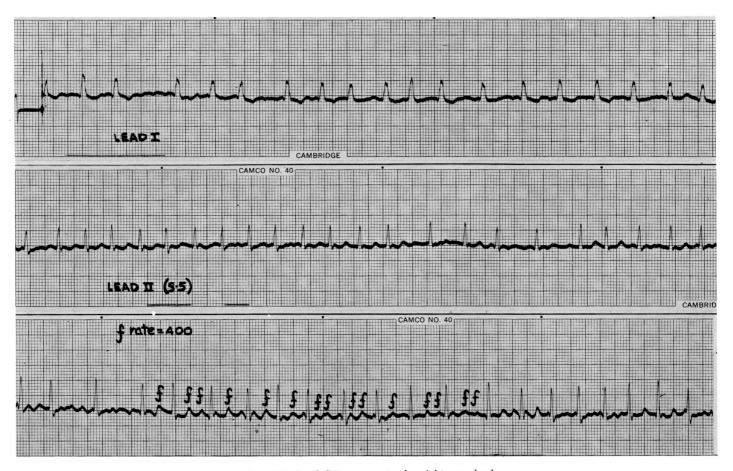

Fig. 4-45. Lead S-5 represents the right arm lead with the suction cup over the manubrium of the sternum and the left arm lead just to the right of the sternum in the fourth or fifth interspace and it is taken as Lead I. This lead accentuates the P wave (atrial or auricular complexes). L-II is taken if lead I is of low voltage. This S-5 lead is also known as the Lewis Lead. It is used to bring out p wave, f and F waves, as in this case of atrial fibrillation.

CHAPTER 5

Premature Ventricular Systoles

Definition: Single or multiple premature QRS beats arising from an ectopic focus somewhere in either ventricle.

ECG Characteristics

Ventricular complex (QRS) is not preceded by a premature P' wave.

Duration of QRS is 0.12 sec. or longer.

The closer the focus of origin is to the bifurcation of the bundle of His, the more the QRS resembles a ventricular complex of sinus or nodal origin.

QRS is bizarre: slurred, notched, bifid, thickened limbs.

P wave rhythm is not interrupted (i.e., the sinus rhythm).

A compensatory pause follows the P.V.C.

T wave is large and moves in opposite direction to major deflection and therefore T wave is negative.

Clinical Significance

1. The wider and the more bizarre the QRS, the more likely the premature ventricular contraction is pathological. (A QRS of 0.18 sec. or more is pathological.)

2. Appearance on exercise makes P.V.C.'s pathologically suspicious of possible myocardial ischemia or coronary artery insufficiency.

3. Disappearance after exercise indicates P.V.C. is innocent.

4. Wide Q waves and depression of ST-T segments showing up only in ventricular extrasystole is indicative of infarction.

5. Negative T waves in the beat follow-

(*Text continues on page 59*)

FIGURE 5-1

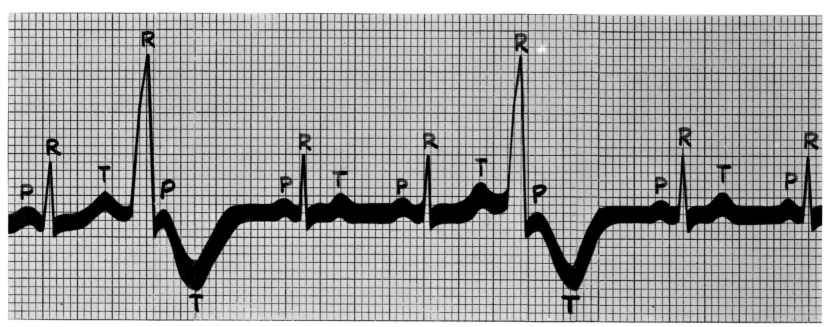

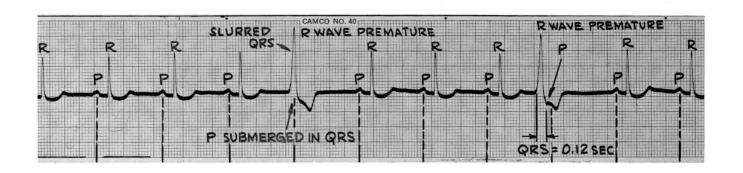

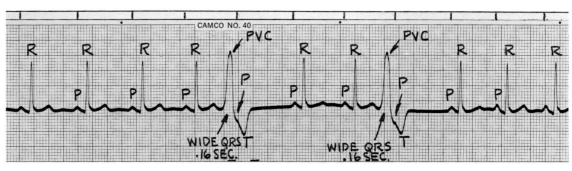

(Top) Fig. 5-2. Ventricular premature contraction (ventricular extrasystoles). Note that the P wave rhythm is uninterrupted.

(Right) Fig. 5-3. Premature ventricular contraction. P wave rhythm is uninterrupted. R wave rhythm is interrupted by premature R waves.

(Bottom) Fig. 5-4. $(R_1 - X)$ plus $(X - R_2)$ equals $2R - R$ intervals. Thus, the P wave rhythm is unaltered.

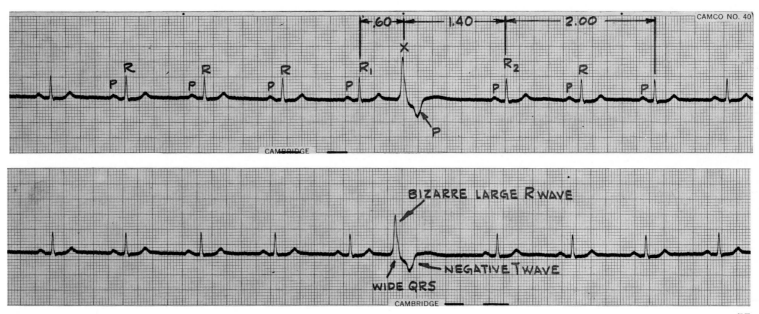

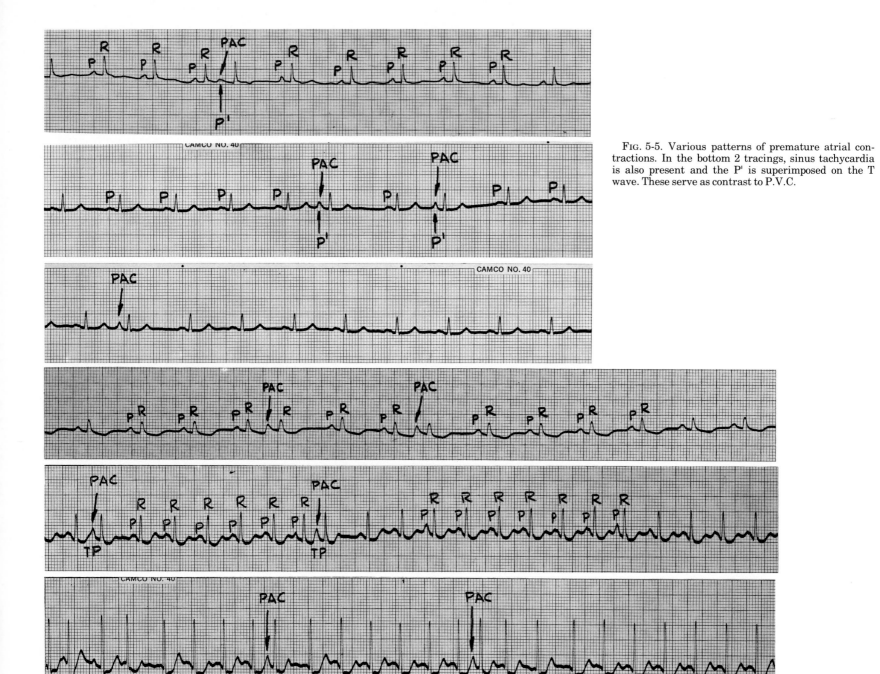

FIG. 5-5. Various patterns of premature atrial contractions. In the bottom 2 tracings, sinus tachycardia is also present and the P' is superimposed on the T wave. These serve as contrast to P.V.C.

ing the ventricular extrasystole are indicative of ischemia.

6. Should the premature ventricular contraction be close to or on the descending limb of the T wave it may hit the vulnerable phase of systole and trigger a ventricular tachycardia.

7. Premature ventricular contractions may be the earliest sign of digitalis intoxication.

8. An increase in the number of P.V.C.'s during a Master's test may be indicative of coronary artery disease with ischemia or insufficiency.

9. In diseased hearts, multifocal or paroxysmal premature ventricular contractions may be the forerunner of ventricular tachycardia or ventricular fibrillation.

Occurrence

Premature ventricular contractions may occur in normal hearts

Precipitating Factors

Emotional stress
Coffee
Tobacco
Drugs
   Quinidine
   Procainamide
   Atropine
   Digitalis
   Nicotine
   Epinephrine
Electrolyte imbalances (e.g., potassium depletion following diuretic therapy)
Cardiac catheterization

CHAPTER 6

Bundle Branch Block

A complete bundle branch block signifies that for some reason conduction through either of the branches of the bundle of His has been delayed or interrupted. This delay or interruption causes a widening of the QRS complex to at least 0.12 sec.

Right bundle branch block or left bundle branch block may occasionally be found in normal hearts.

Conditions Associated with Left or Right Bundle Branch Block (or Bundle Branch Block Patterns)

Congenital heart disease
    Atrial septal defect
    Pulmonary stenosis
Rheumatic heart disease, especially calcific aortic stenosis and mitral stenosis
Coronary artery disease
Coronary atherosclerosis
Myocardial infarction
Hypertensive heart disease
Infectious diseases
    Diphtheria
    Bacterial endocarditis
    Virus infections
    Syphilis (syphilitic aortic incompetence)
    Chronic myocarditis
Iatrogenic factors, especially during cardiac surgery
Drugs
    Excessive potassium intake, especially of the recently developed potassium salt products

(*Text continues on page 69*)

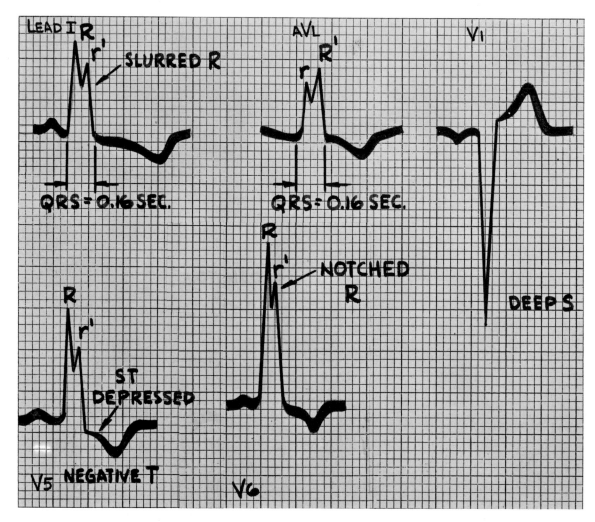

FIG. 6-1. Left bundle branch block—complete. Note M pattern in V5 and V6. (ECG criteria for left bundle branch block, complete, see p. 69.)

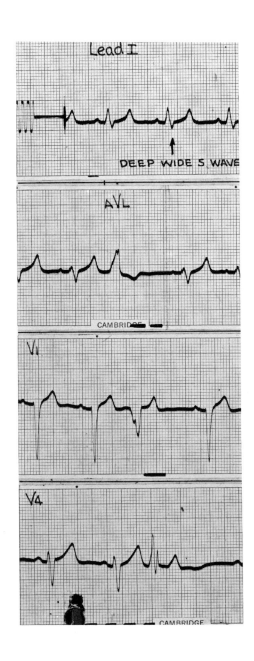

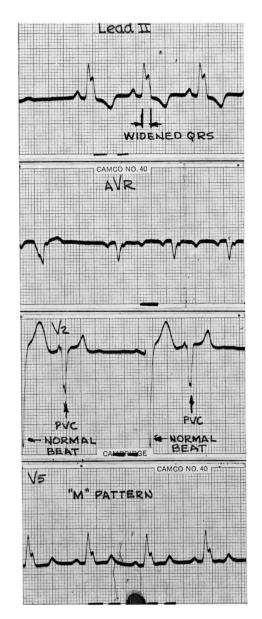

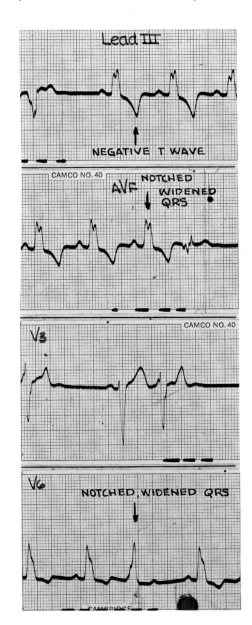

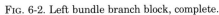

FIG. 6-2. Left bundle branch block, complete.

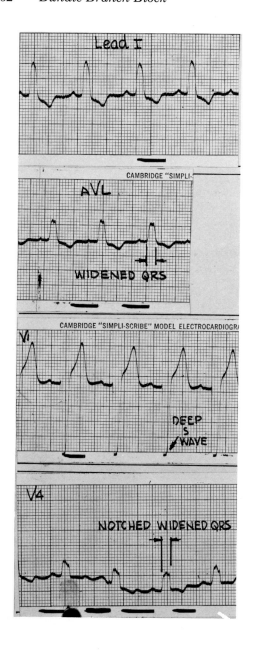
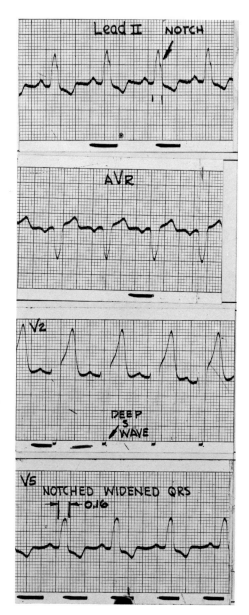
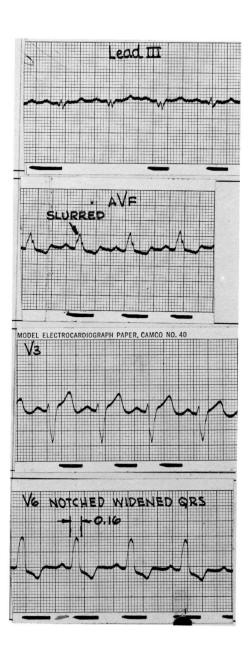

FIG. 6-3. Left bundle branch block, complete.

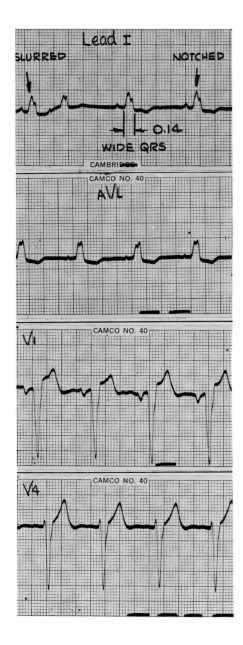
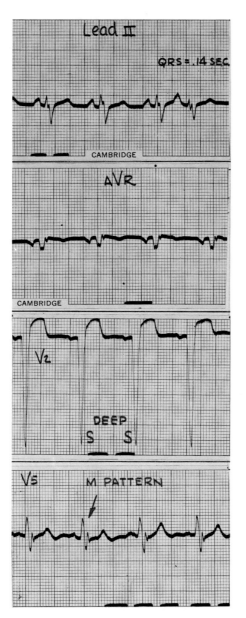
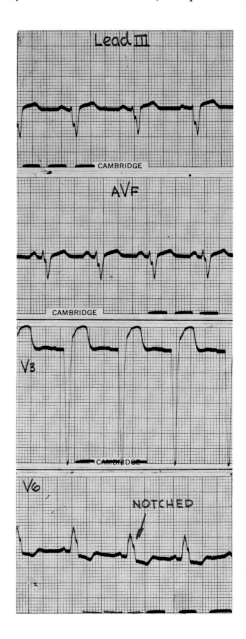

FIG. 6-4. Left bundle branch block, complete.

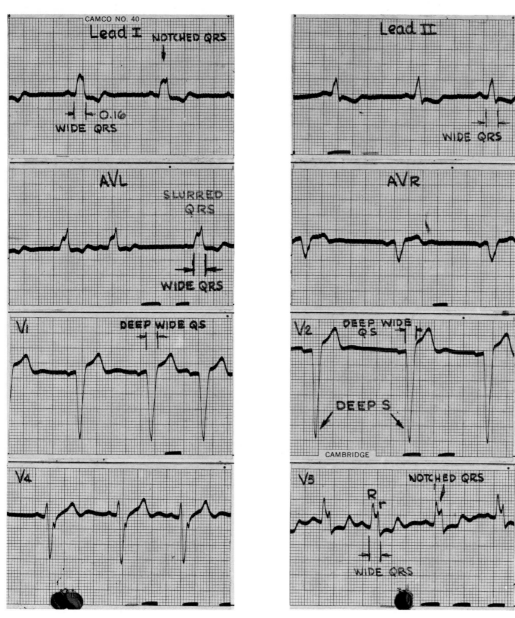
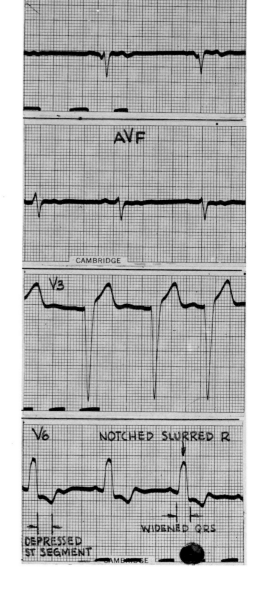

FIG. 6-5. Left bundle branch block, complete.

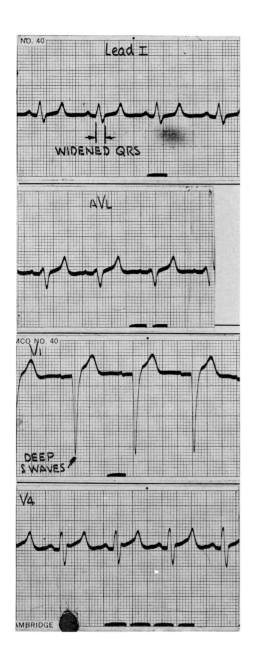
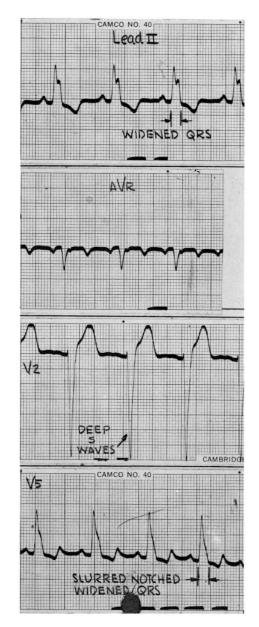
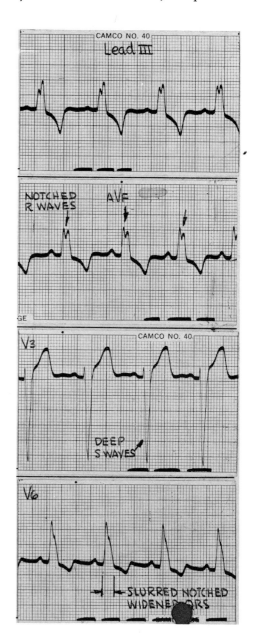

Fig. 6-6. Left bundle branch block, complete.

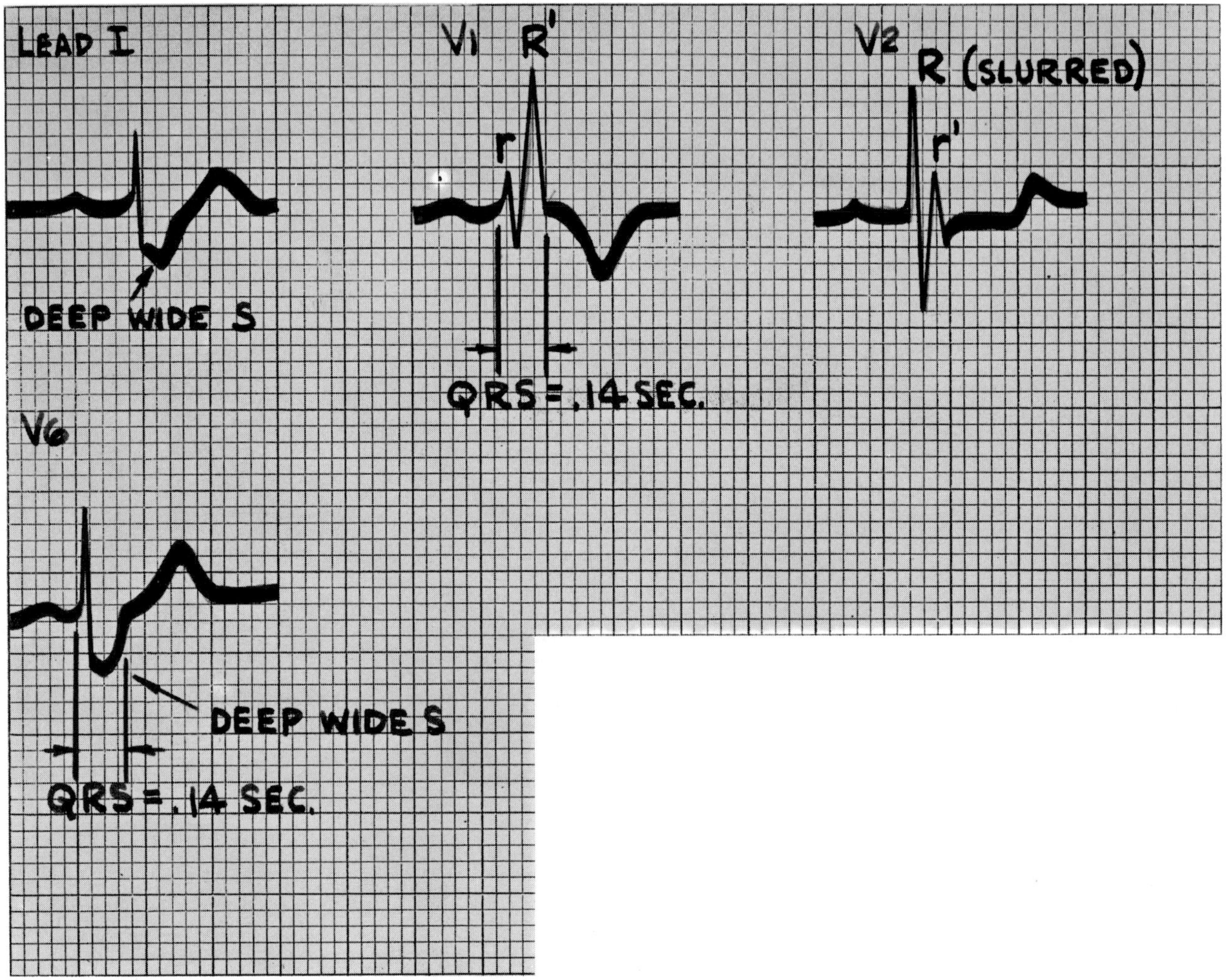

FIG. 6-7. Complete right bundle branch block. Note M pattern in V₁ and V₂. See page 69 for ECG criteria.

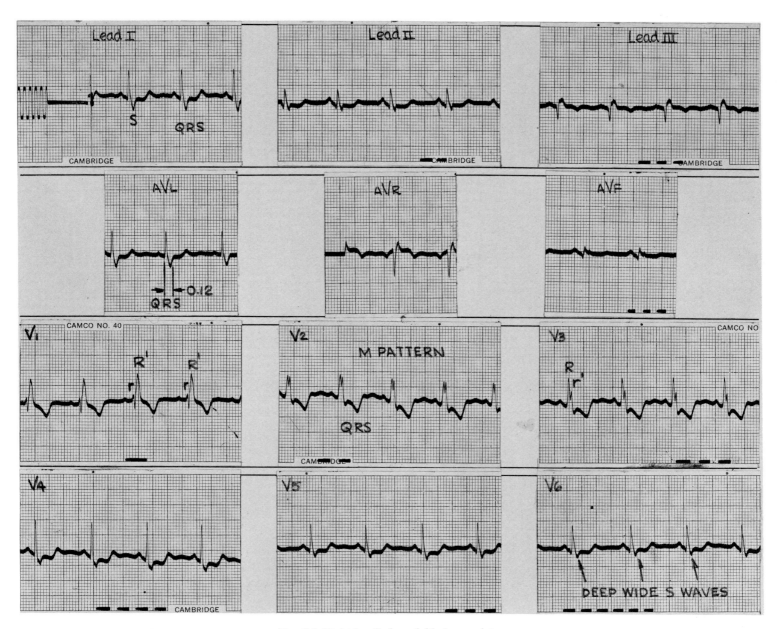

F1G. 6-8. Right bundle branch block, complete.

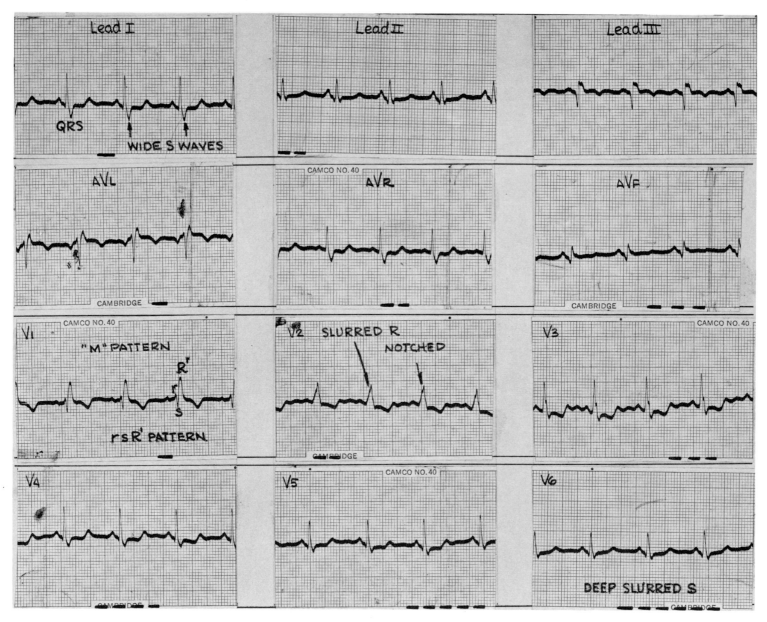

FIG. 6-9. Right bundle branch block, complete.

Quinidine
Procainamide
Digitalis

Tachycardia such as paroxysmal atrial tachycardia may cause fatigue of the bundle and, therefore, prolongation of the QRS interval.

Complete Left Bundle Branch Block

Electrocardiographic Criteria (Fig. 6-1)

1. The QRS complexes must be 0.12 sec. or greater.

2. The QRS is slurred and notched; the T wave usually is inscribed in the opposite direction to the R wave in almost all leads.

3. The W pattern is seen in V_1 and V_2; the M pattern in V_5 and/or V_6.

4. The intrinsicoid deflection (known also as ventricular activation time—V.A.T.) in V_4, V_5, or V_6 is delayed at least 0.04 sec. to 0.05 sec.

Figures 6-2 to 6-6 are examples of left bundle branch block patterns.

Complete Right Bundle Branch Block

Electrocardiographic Criteria (Fig. 6-7)

1. Usually shows right axis deviation
2. QRS greater than 0.12 sec.
3. Wide and slurred S wave in leads I, V_5 and V_6.
4. rsR′ pattern in V_1 and V_2 (M pattern in V_2 or V_3) and deep wide S wave in V_5 and V_6. V.A.T. = 0.06 sec. or longer.
5. Normal continuity of PQRST relationship

Figures 6-8 through 6-10 are examples of the patterns typical of complete right bundle branch block.

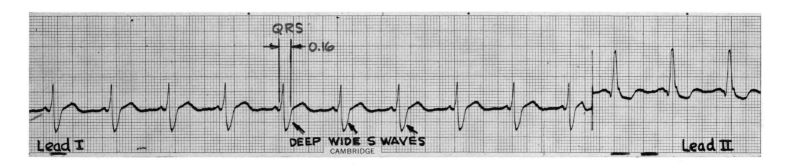

FIG. 6-10. Right bundle branch block, complete.

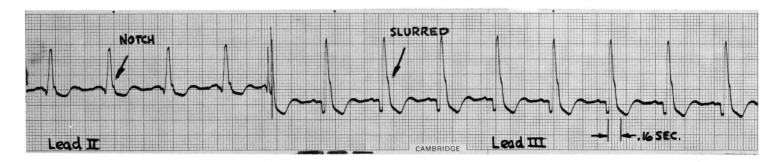

CHAPTER 7

Ventricular Hypertrophy

Left Ventricular Hypertrophy

Definition: Enlargement of the left ventricle through increase in weight and mass of myocardial tissue, with stretching of the muscle fibers.

Causes

Congenital heart disease
    Interventricular septal defect
    Aortic or subaortic stenosis
    Patent ductus arteriosus
    Endocardial fibroelastosis
Rheumatic heart disease
Hypertensive heart disease
Coronary artery disease
Nutritional
    Beriberi
    Anemia
    Chronic alcoholism
Endocrine disorders
    Hyperthyroidism
    Hypothyroidism (myxedema)

ECG Criteria

I. *Standard limb leads* (Fig. 7-1)

1. Voltage R_1 plus voltage S_3 is 25 mm. or greater.

2. RS-T_1 depressed 0.5 mm. or more; negative T_1, or T_1 and T_2 — ventricular strain.

3. T_1 flat, diphasic or inverted, particularly when T_1, or T_1 and T_2 are associated with depressed RS-T segment and R_1 is prominent and upright (+25 mm. or more).

4. T_2 and T_3 diphasic or inverted in the presence of tall R waves and depressed RS-T segment in a vertical heart.

5. T_3 has greater amplitude than T_1 in the presence of left axis deviation, high voltage QRS in lead I, and deep S_3 wave.

6. Left axis deviation, usually.

Fig. 7-1. Left ventricular hypertrophy, standard limb leads.

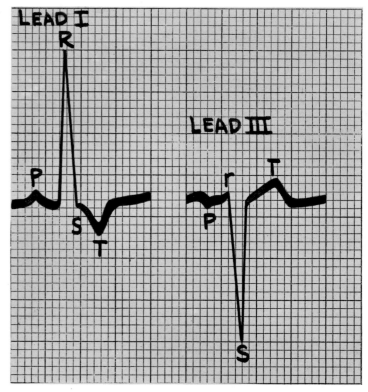

II. *Precordial leads* (Fig. 7-2)

1. Voltage of R wave in V_5 or V_6 exceeds 26 mm.

2. RS-T segment depressed more than 0.5 mm. in V_4, V_5 or V_6.

3. RS-T may be elevated 2 mm. in V_1, V_2, V_3. If this appears in all precordial leads in serial electrocardiograms, it is diagnostic of persistent ventricular aneurysm.

4. Flat, diphasic or inverted T wave in leads V_4 through V_6, normal R, small s waves, and depressed RS-T (more than 0.5 mm.) in V_4, V_5 or V_6.

5. SV_1 plus $SV_2 > 30$ mm.
   RV_5 plus $RV_6 > 30$ mm.

6. SV_2 plus $RV_5 > 35$ mm.

7. U wave > mm.

8. RV_6 taller than RV_5.

III. *Unipolar limb leads* (Fig. 7-3)

1. Voltage of R wave in aVL exceeds 11.0 mm. in a transverse heart.

2. RS-T segment depressed more than 0.5 mm. in aVL or aVF.

3. Upright T wave in aVR.

4. R wave amplitudes 21 mm. or more in aVF—vertical heart.

(*Text continues on p. 76*)

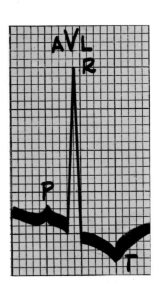

Fig. 7-3. Left ventricular hypertrophy. Unipolar limb lead.

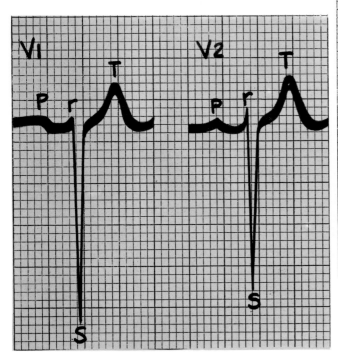

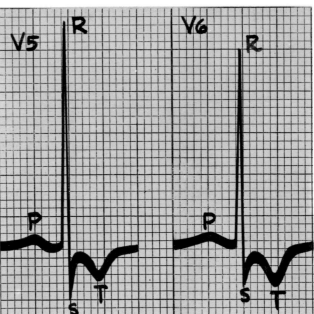

Fig. 7-2. Left ventricular hypertrophy (precordial leads).

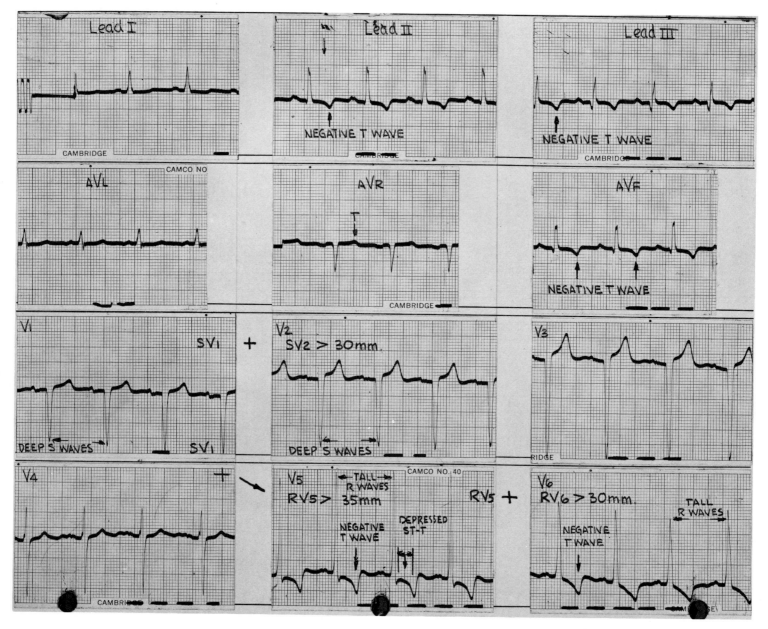

FIG. 7-4. Left ventricular hypertrophy.

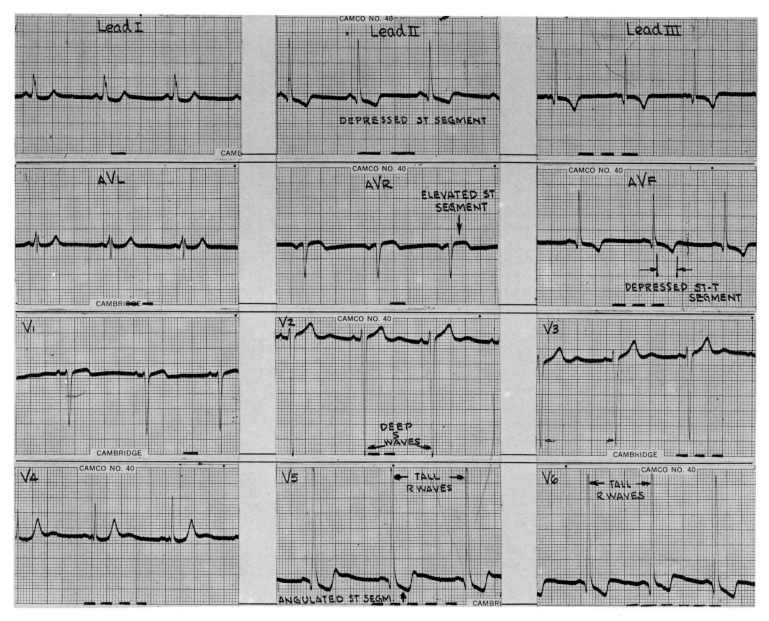

Fig. 7-5. Left ventricular hypertrophy and digitalis effect.

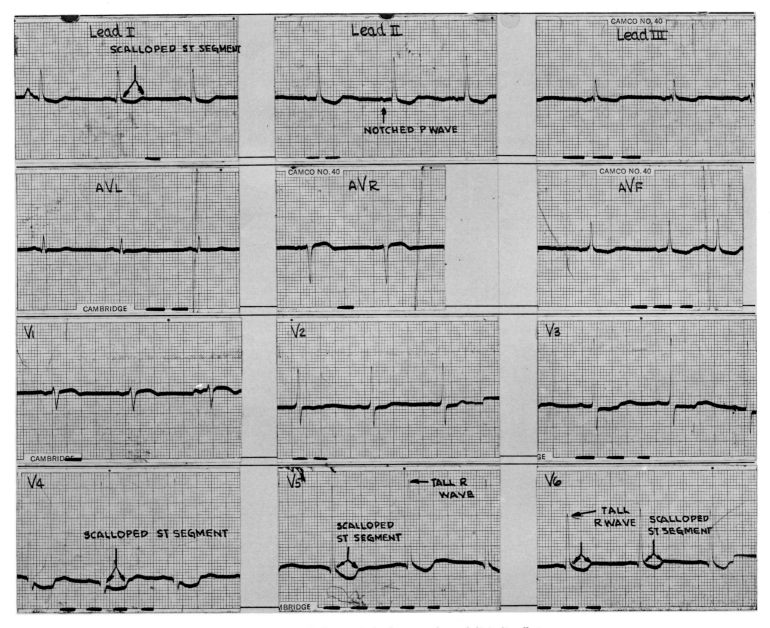

Fig. 7-6. Left ventricular hypertrophy and digitalis effect.

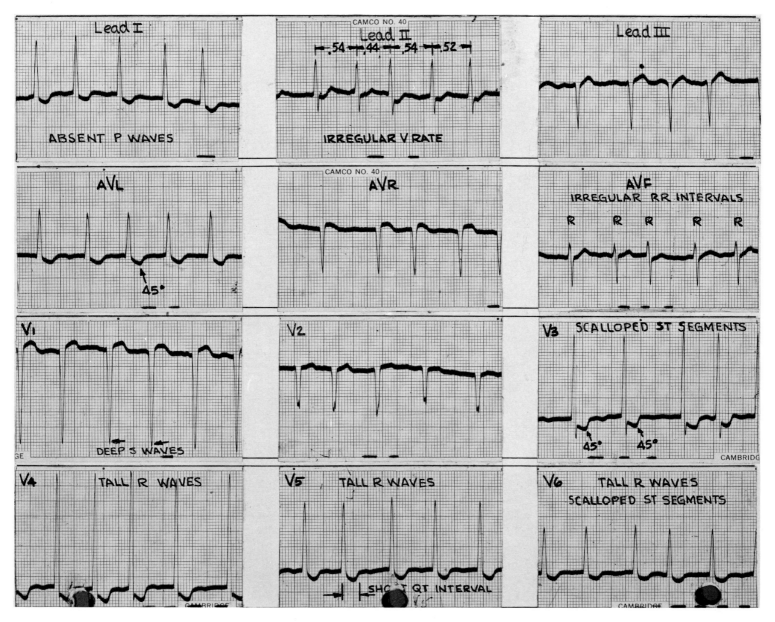

F_IG. 7-7. Left ventricular hypertrophy, digitalis effect, and atrial fibrillation.

Right Ventricular Hypertrophy

Right ventricular hypertrophy is enlargement of the right ventricle.

Occurrence

Mitral stenosis
Congenital heart disease
Atrial septal defect
Pulmonary stenosis
Tetralogy of Fallot
Pulmonary arterial disease
Pulmonary embolism, recurrent
Chronic cor pulmonale

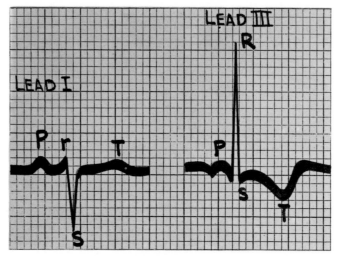

Figure 7-8

Figure 7-10. (*below*)

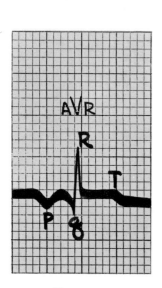

Figure 7-9

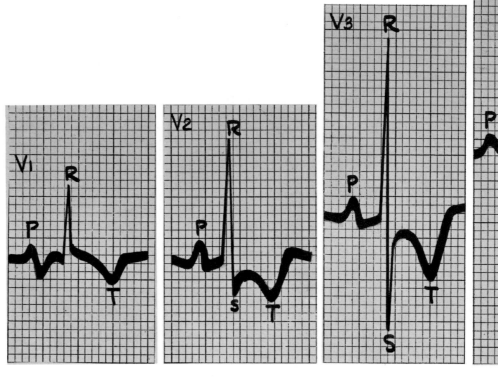

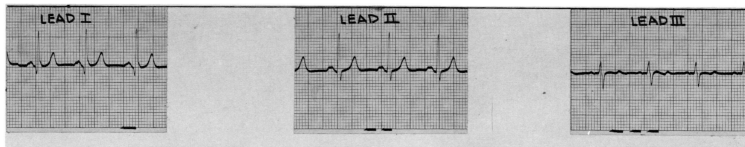

ECG Criteria

I. *Standard leads* (Fig. 7-8)

1. Right axis deviation, +90° to 180°, +180° to −90°. S in lead I is deep; R in lead III is upward.

2. The sum of the voltages of S_1 and R_3 is greater than 25 mm.

3. S-T in leads II and III depressed 0.5 mm. or more.

4. P waves notched or peaked (p pulmonale).

5. T_2 and T_3 may be negative (25% of cases).

II. *Unipolar limb leads* (Fig. 7-9)

1. aVR: R > 4 mm.

III. *Precordial leads* (Fig. 7-10)

1. RV_1 large, S absent. RV_1 or V_3R is greater than 7 mm.

2. Ascending limb of RV_1 is 0.035 sec. or more (intrinsicoid deflection). Q wave often present in V_1.

3. R in V_6 peaks at 0.02 sec. (early intrinsicoid deflection).

4. Negative T in V_1, V_2, or all precordial leads.

5. Rr' or rR' pattern in V_1 or V_2.
   R/S ratio in $V_1 > 1$
   R/S ratio in $V_6 < 1$

6. Right bundle branch block pattern may be found.

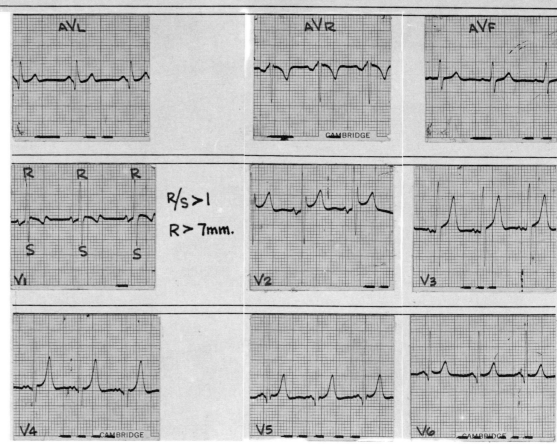

Fig. 7-11. Right ventricular hypertrophy. Note in V_1, R/S > 1; R > 7 mm.

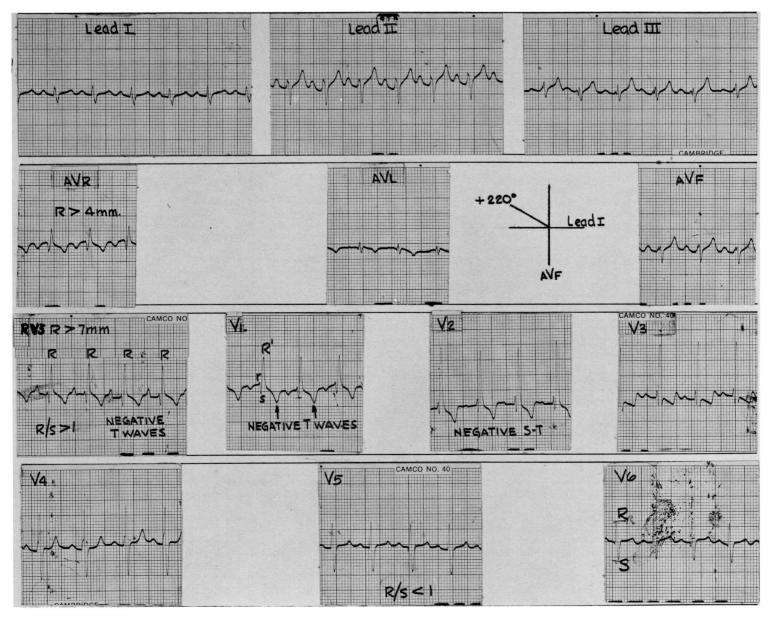

FIG. 7-12. Right ventricular hypertrophy. Note R_1BBB pattern in V_2 and V_3.

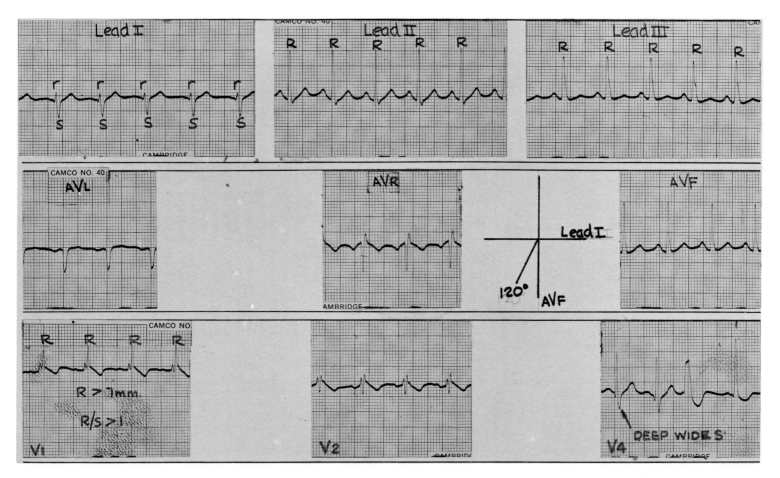

F<small>IG</small>. 7-13. Right ventricular hypertrophy.

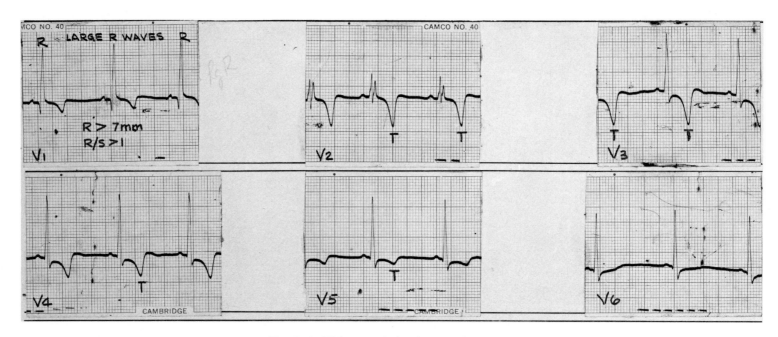

FIG. 7-14. Right ventricular hypertrophy. Precordial leads.

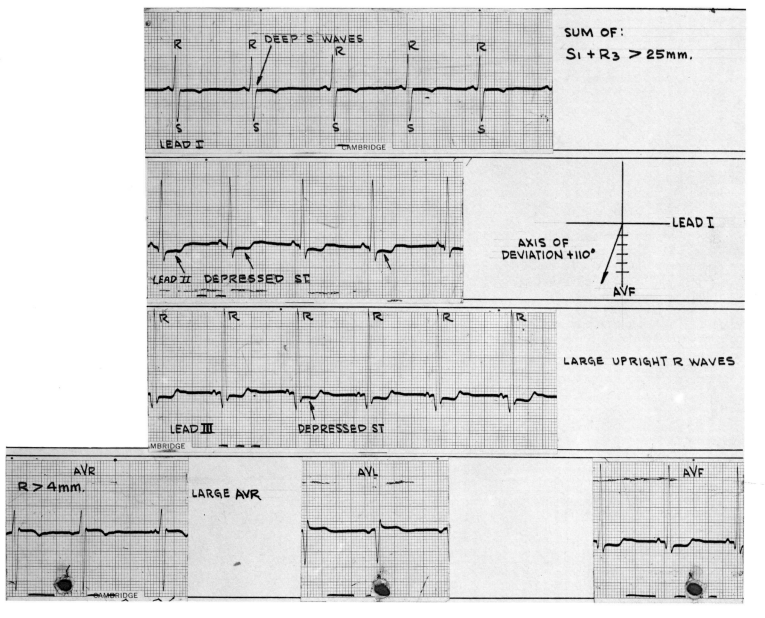

FIG. 7-15. Right ventricular hypertrophy. Standard
and aV leads. Note that the sum of S₁ and R₃ is greater
than 25 mm. R waves in lead III are very tall.

CHAPTER 8

Nodal Rhythm

Nodal rhythm arises in the atrioventricular node, either by usurpation or by default of the S-A pacemaking function.

Anatomically, the A-V node is a small, oval neuromuscular structure, measuring about 6 mm. x 3 mm. It is located in the upper part of the heart to the right of the crux (cross of the heart), adjacent to the central fibrous body (i.e., the intersection of the atrial and the ventricular septa). The upper portion of the node arises near the coronary sinus in the right atrium.

The A-V node is composed of three sections:

1. The upper portion (the A-N section): in this section there are pacemaker fibers.

2. The midportion (the N section): in this section there are no pacemaker fibers.

3. The lower portion (the N-H section, or nodal His section): it is from this site that most of the A-V nodal rhythms originate.

The A-V node is supplied by a small artery called the ramus septi fibrosi. This small branch is supplied in about 90 per cent of hearts by the right coronary artery. Therefore, lesions of the posterior coronary arteries (branches of the right coronary artery) frequently cause A-V block and nodal rhythms.

In a true nodal rhythm the P wave is always positive in aVR. It may precede or follow the QRS complex or lie within it.

The function of the A-V node, which possesses inherent rhythmicity, is to conduct impulses, anterograde or retrograde. A-V node can take over command in the following ways:

1. By default, to produce passive escape rhythm.

2. By active rhythm: accelerated nonparoxysmal nodal tachycardia, analogous to sinus tachycardia. The rate is 70 to 150.

3. By paroxysmal nodal rhythm. The rate is 150 to 250.

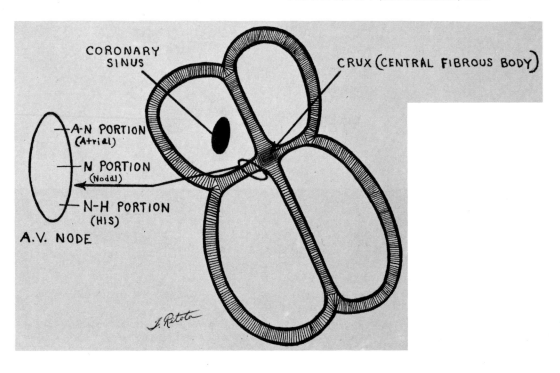

Fig. 8-1. The A-V (atrioventricular) node.

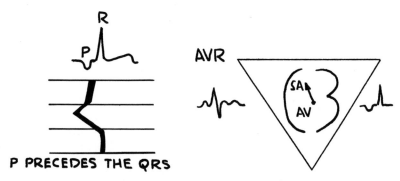

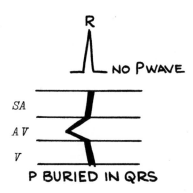

FIG. 8-2. Upper nodal rhythm. Note the characteristics of the nodal P wave. (*Left*) Duration of P is less than 0.12 sec. P wave is inverted because the impulse travels from the node upward. (*Right*) P is diphasic or flat in lead I, negative in leads II and III, and upright in aVR.

FIG. 8-3. Middle nodal rhythm. There is simultaneous stimulation of the atria and the ventricles, and the P wave is buried in the ventricular complex.

A wandering pacemaker is common in A-V nodal rhythm (the pacemaker shifting back and forth from the S-A (sinus pacemaker) node to the A-V node).

Nodal rhythm may have a prolonged P-R interval, but usually the P-R interval is shorter than normal. In 80 per cent of A-V nodal rhythms, the P waves occur before the QRS complexes.

Nodal escape beats are rare without interference. When the P wave is upright in lead II and the P-R interval is less than 0.10 sec., the P wave really originates from the sinus node and the ventricular complex

from the A-V node. This shows interference with nodal beat. This is known as interference dissociation.

Causes

    Digitalis intoxication (most common)
    Rheumatic fever with myocarditis
    Acute infections
    Vagal normal rhythms
    Posterior wall infarctions
  Digitalis increases the rhythmicity of all ectopic foci. Reciprocal rhythms are encountered in nodal rhythms.

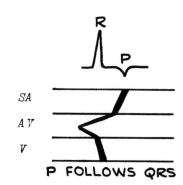

FIG. 8-4. Lower nodal rhythm. The ventricles are stimulated before the atria; therefore the ventricular complex is written first. The atrial P wave that follows is retrograde (inverted).

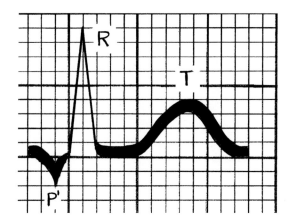

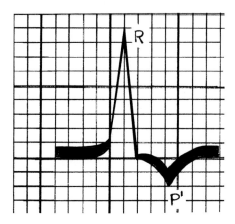

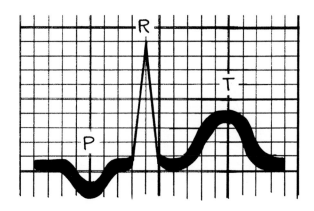

P—NODAL BEFORE THE R WAVE.

P—NODAL AFTER THE R WAVE.

NORMAL NEGATIVE P WAVE OR LEFT AURICULAR P WAVE (FOUND IN LEAD I).

FIG. 8-5. Forms of nodal P waves. (*Left*) The P wave is inverted, sharply peaked, narrow (resembling an arrow). Duration about 0.08 sec. (less than 0.10 sec.). (*Center*) Inverted, sharply peaked P wave following the QRS. (*Right*) The P wave is negative but has a normal P-R interval and is not sharply peaked.

The P-R interval of nodal beats is about 0.10 seconds or less. P is flat in lead I, negative in leads II, III and aVF, and upright in aVR and aVL.

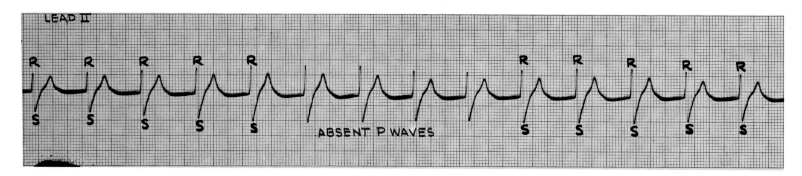

FIG. 8-6. Nodal rhythm. Note that R-R intervals are regular. P waves are submerged in RS.

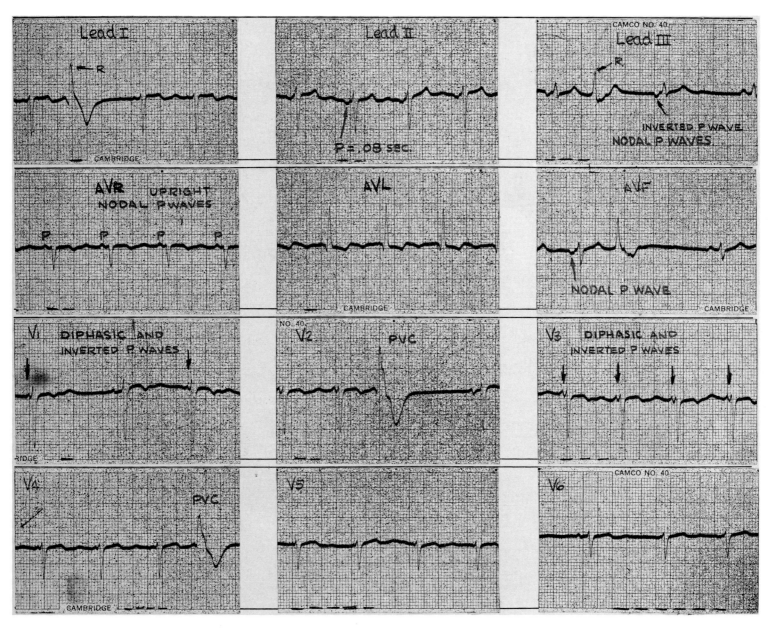

Fig. 8-7. Premature ventricular contraction, nodal
P waves and nodal rhythm. Nodal beats precede QRS.

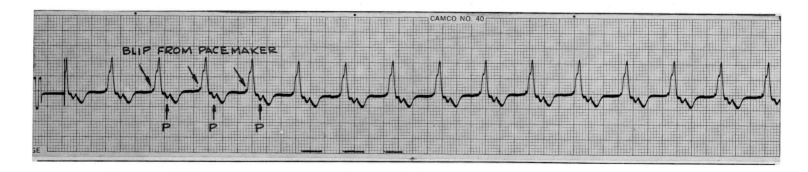

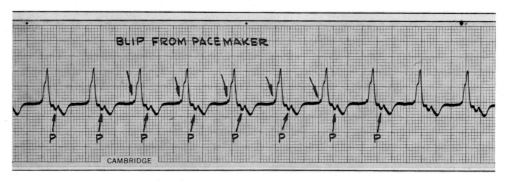

FIG. 8-8. Nodal P waves. Note spikes from pacemaker.
Nodal beats follow QRS.

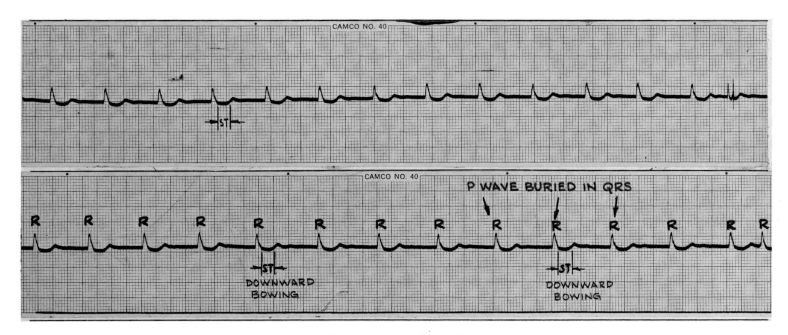

Fɪɢ. 8-9. Nodal rhythm and digitalis effect. R-R
rhythm is regular, with rate of 70. Note that P waves
are not discernible: Nodal P waves are submerged in
the R waves.

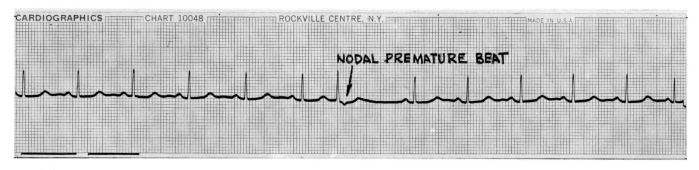

Fɪɢ. 8-10. Nodal premature beat. P follows QRS and
is retrograde (inverted). Complex is narrow.

CHAPTER 9

Heart Block

First Degree Heart Block
(Prolonged P-R Interval; A-V Nodal Delay)

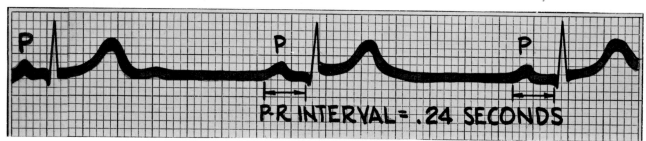

FIGURE 9-1

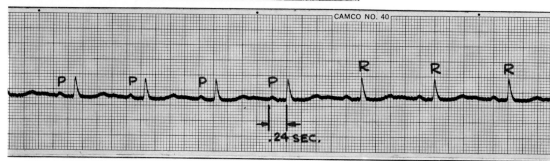

FIG. 9-2. Prolonged P-R interval in first degree heart block. Normal P-R interval is 0.20 sec. In this tracing the P-R interval is 0.24 sec.

Definition: First degree heart block, or A-V nodal delay, is delay in conduction of the impulse, after its origin in the S-A node and spread through the atria, in the atrio-ventricular node, resulting in increase in conduction time of the impulse from the S-A node to the ventricular muscle.

First degree heart block may be a congenital condition.

Conditions Associated with First Degree Heart Block

Rheumatic fever
Coronary artery disease
Arteriosclerotic heart disease
Acute posterior wall infarction
Digitalis excess

ECG Criteria

Prolonged P-R interval: longer than 0.20 sec. in adults (varies with heart rate)
Normal P waves
Normal QRS
Regular sinus rhythm

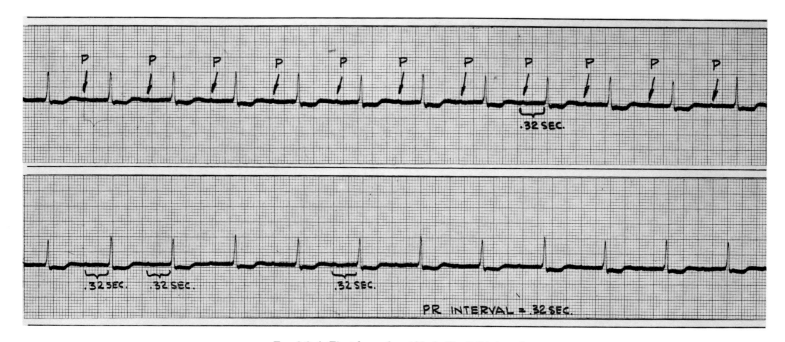

FIG. 9-3. A. First degree heart block. The P-R interval
is prolonged to 0.32 sec. (normal, 0.20 sec.).

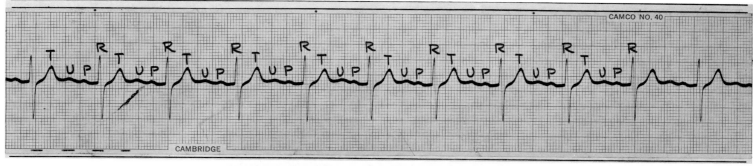

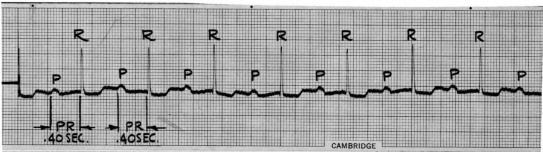

FIG. 9-3. (B) Prolonged P-R interval, P-R = 0.24
(normal P-R for this rate—0.20 to 0.21). U waves are
clearly seen. (C) Prolonged P-R interval in first degree
heart block (A-V nodal delay). (Normal P-R for this
rate is 0.20–0.21.) P–QRS relationship is constant,
indicating sinus rhythm.

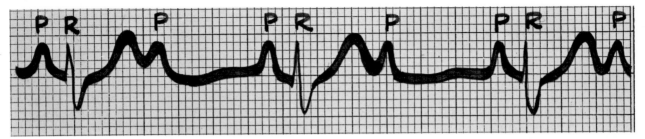

FIG. 9-4. Second degree atrioventricular block.

Second Degree Atrioventricular Block

When the impulses originating in the sinoauricular node and passing through the atria arrive at the atrioventricular node, every second, third or fourth beat may be conducted (2:1 block; 3:1 block; 4:1 block) or may be blocked (3:2 block; 4:3 block).

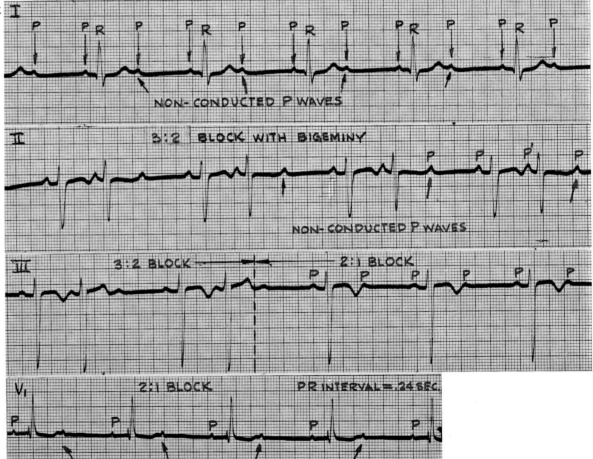

FIG. 9-5. Second degree heart block. Rate of P waves is 85 per min. Rate of R waves is 40 per min. Lead I is 2:1 heart block. Lead II arrows indicate nonconducted P waves.

**Conditions Associated With
Second Degree Heart Block**

Rheumatic heart disease
Coronary artery disease
Digitalis effect
Quinidine effect

ECG Criteria

The ventricular rate is slower than the atrial rate, commonly in the ratio of 1:2, 1:3, or 1:4.
Normal P waves
Normal QRS complexes
QRS is written usually only after every second, third or fourth P wave
QRS may fail to appear only after third or fourth P wave

**Complete Heart Block
(Third Degree A-V Block)**

Definition. Complete heart block is an arrhythmia in which none of the impulses arising in the sinoatrial node and passing through the atria is conducted through the atrioventricular node to the bundle or its branches. The pacemaker for the ventricles is located either in the A-V node or below it (in the ventricle). Thus, the ventricular rhythm, which may be *idioventricular* or *idionodal*, is independent of the atrial rhythm.

**Conditions Associated With
Complete Heart Block**

Rheumatic heart disease
Diphtheria
Congenital heart disease
Cardiac surgery
Digitalis toxicity
Coronary artery disease
Acute coronary thrombosis, posterior wall type

ECG Criteria

1. The atrial and the ventricular rhythms are absolutely independent of one another.
2. There is no P-R to QRS relationship.
3. The atrial rate is more rapid than the ventricular rate.
4. The atrial rate is not a constant multiple of the ventricular rate.
5. *Idioventricular rhythm*
   QRS is 0.12 sec. or greater.
   QRS is bizarre, slurred and notched.
   Idioventricular rate is 36 beats per min. or less.
6. *Idionodal rhythm*
   QRS is less than 0.12 sec.
   QRS complexes are normal in shape.
   Ventricular rate is 36 to 40 beats per min.

FIGURES 9-7 through 9-9 follow on pages 92-94.

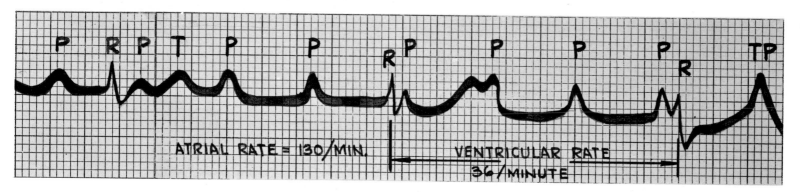

FIGURE 9-6

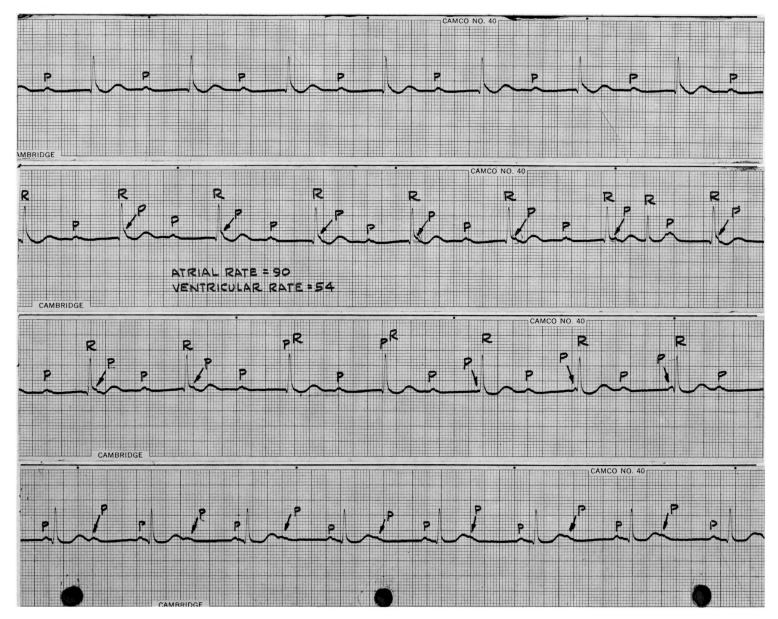

FIG. 9-7. Complete heart block (third degree heart block). Idionodal type.

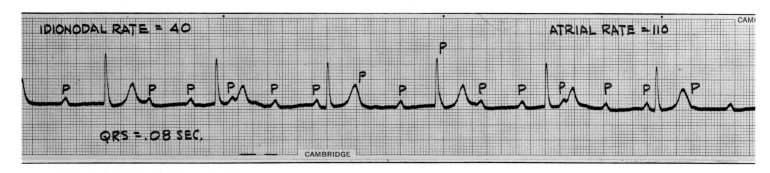

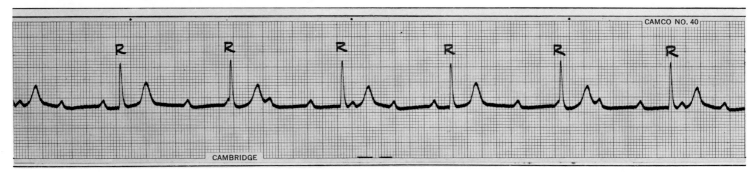

FIG. 9-8. Complete heart block: idionodal rhythm.

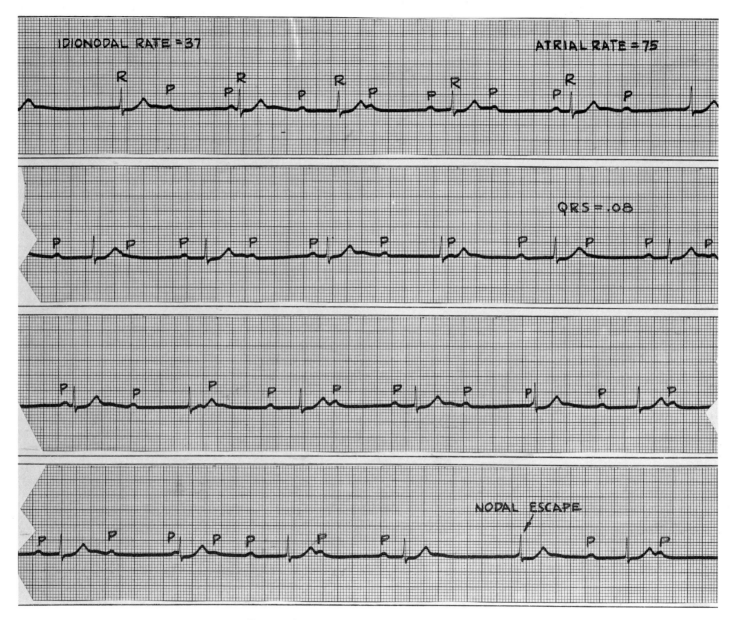

FIG. 9-9. Complete heart block: idionodal rhythm.

CHAPTER 10

Acute Pericarditis

Acute Pericarditis

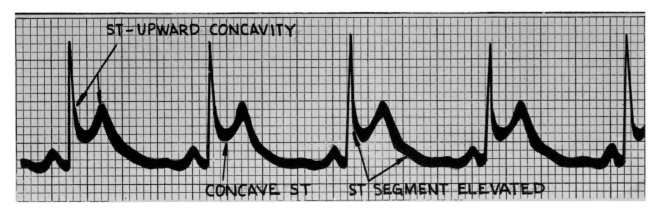

FIGURE 10-1

Definition: Acute pericarditis is an inflammatory process of the visceral or parietal pericardium.

Conditions Associated With Acute Pericarditis

Rheumatic fever
Infarction
Uremia
Pyogenic infections
Tuberculosis
Malignancies
Collagen disease

ECG Criteria*

S-T changes occur within first 24 hours
S-T segment elevated one to three mm.
ST—shows an upward concavity
T vector variable from day to day
No QRS abnormalities
S-T returns to the isoelectric line
T wave becomes negative
No pathological Q wave
No reciprocal S-T changes in lead I and lead III.

* Hurst, J. W., et al.: Electrocardiographic Interpretation. pp. 209, 212. New York, McGraw-Hill, 1963.

FIG. 10-2. (*Top*) Early acute pericarditis. Upward concavity: The S-T segment is slightly elevated, T wave is elevated and upright.

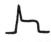

FIG. 10-2. (*Bottom*) Early acute infarction. Upward convexity: S-T segment is elevated.

95

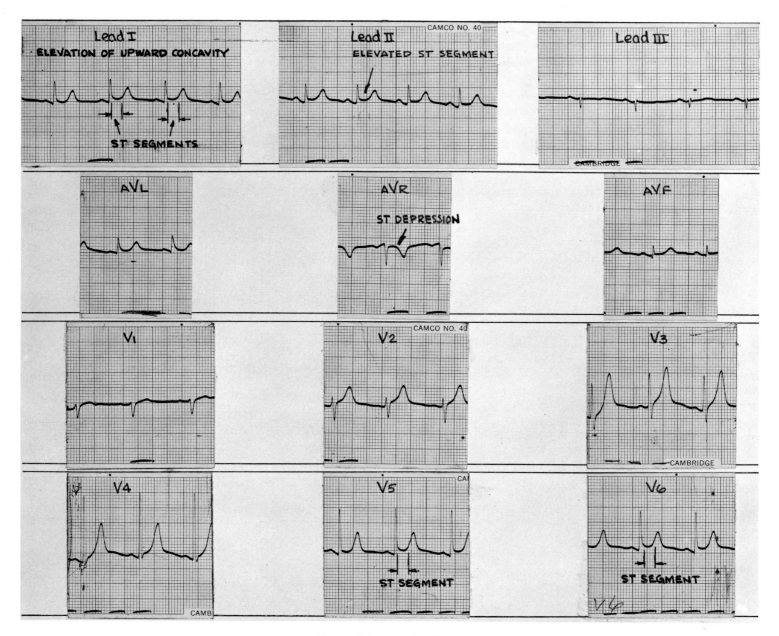

Fig. 10-3. Acute pericarditis.

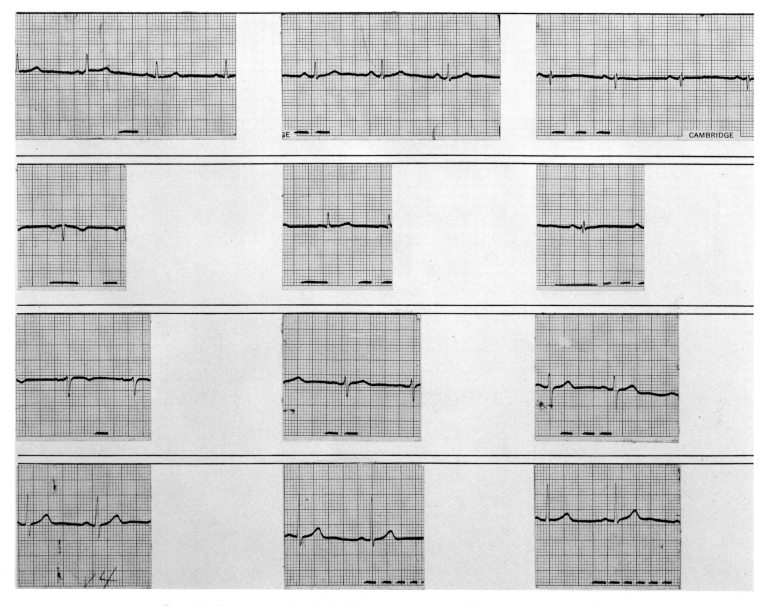

Fig. 10-4. Same case as Fig. 10-3, ECG taken several days later. Note ST has returned to isoelectric line in leads I, II, V_5 and V_6.

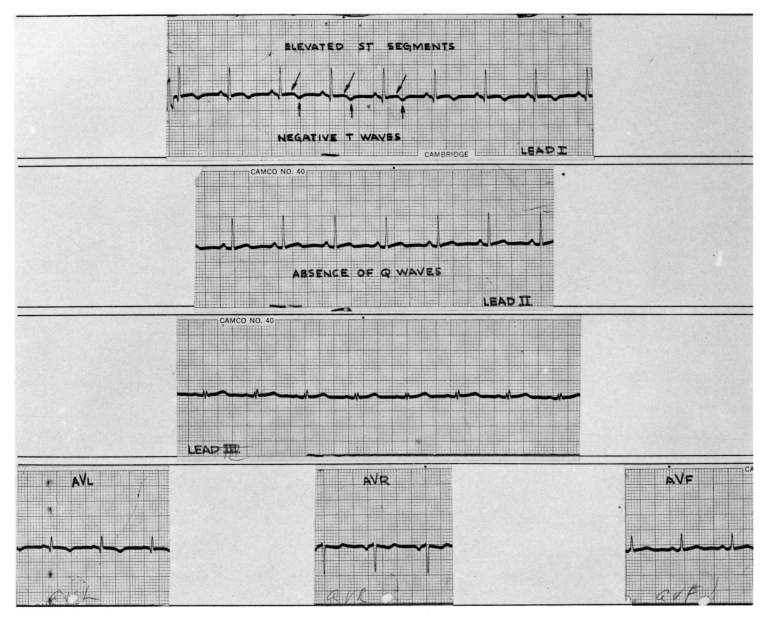

FIG. 10-5. Acute pericarditis. Significant diagnostic
features are: absence of Q waves; elevation of S-T segment; negative T waves.

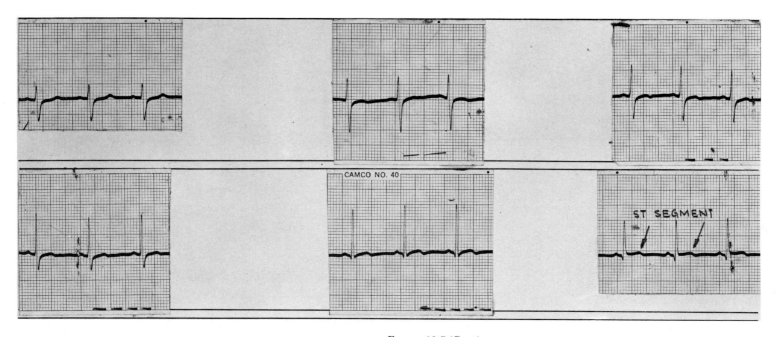

FIGURE 10-5 *(Cont.)*

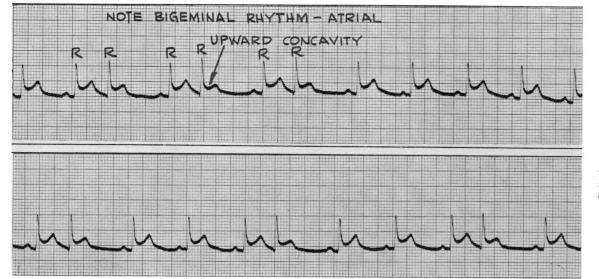

FIG. 10-6. Strip from ECG lead II from patient with acute pericarditis. Compare with Figure 10-7, also lead II, showing pattern typical of acute myocardial infarction.

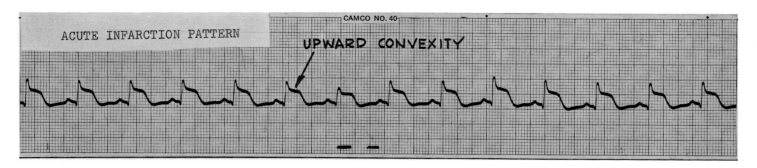

ACUTE INFARCTION PATTERN

CAMCO NO. 40

UPWARD CONVEXITY

FIGURE 10-7

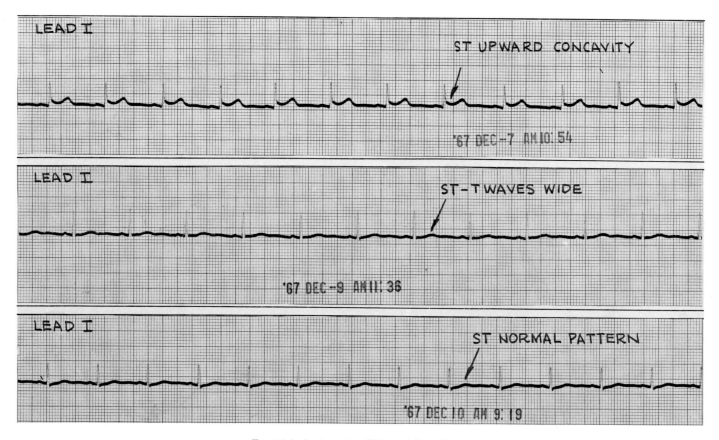

LEAD I

ST UPWARD CONCAVITY

'67 DEC-7 AM 10:54

LEAD I

ST-T WAVES WIDE

'67 DEC-9 AM 11:36

LEAD I

ST NORMAL PATTERN

'67 DEC 10 AM 9:19

FIG. 10-8. Acute pericarditis, serial tracings.

CHAPTER 11

Myocardial Infarction

Recognizing the Candidate for Coronary Heart Disease*

During the winter of 1705 to 1706, Rome was thrown into a state of near panic when one after another of its prominent citizens was struck dead, apparently without warning and in the prime of life. Only one explanation seemed logical to the public: surely God must be angry with Rome! Pope Clement XI and his gifted physician, Lancisi, contested this explanation, and Lancisi proved by post-mortem examinations that even sudden deaths can be due to natural causes. His famous book on sudden deaths, *De Subitaneis Mortibus*, was dedicated to Pope Clement in 1707. In it is quoted this astute and modern-sounding clinical observation, made by Celsus nearly 2,000 years ago, which is certainly applicable today but still generally unheeded:

"No one will have any doubts but that indications of a sudden death ought also to be deduced from an athletic constitution, whenever such athletic persons shall become ever more obese through a sumptuous table, through sleep, and leisure. This very plump and more colorful condition of the body Celsus rightly called a questionable advantage . . . ."

From antiquity, some medical writers have been aware that bad habits of gluttony, idleness, alcoholism, and other excesses presage poor health, and that heredity plays an important role in disease. . . .

There can be no doubt but that coronary heart disease has reached epidemic propor-

*White, P.D.: Consultant, 5:44, 1965.

tions in the United States where it is now responsible for more than 50% of all deaths.

Epidemiology of Myocardial Infarction

Myocardial infarction is more prevalent among Occidentals.

It is more common in countries with a dairy economy.

Incidence is highest in December and January.

Occurrence after unusual physical exertion is relatively rare (7 to 10% of cases).

Time of occurrence is usually about two hours after a heavy meal.

The Predisposed Candidate

The following factors appear to be associated with the occurrence of myocardial infarction!

Sex—male

Build—mesomorphic

Height—below average (about 5' 5")

Age—between 40 and 60 years (50 to 54 critical)

Family history—cardiovascular disease; diabetes; gout; hypertensive heart disease; coronary artery disease

Weight—gain of 25 lbs. in 5 years

Heavy smoker (2 to 3 packs daily)

Etiology of Myocardial Infarction

Myocardial infarction is associated primarily with coronary artery disease. It is caused usually by thrombotic or embolic episodes. Thrombus formation seems to be closely related to atherosclerosis.

Research points to a correlation between diet and the formation of atherosclerotic plaques. It has been found that the death rate from heart disease is comparatively high in groups consuming a diet containing 40 per cent or more of fat, and is low in groups with diets containing 20 per cent or less of fat. Cholesterol appears to be a significant factor and, recently, triglycerides also have been indicated to play a role in atherosclerosis.

Alternatively, the hypothesis has been advanced that thrombus formation is related to fibrin deposition.

Anatomic Factors

The anterior descending branches of the left coronary artery supply the left apex.

The right coronary artery and the left circumflex artery supply the posterior and the lateral wall of the left ventricle.

Thus, thromboembolic episodes or occlusive events, as would be expected, may cause infarction in the area supplied by the artery involved—the left apex, in the case of the former; the posterior or lateral wall, in the case of the latter.

Pathologic Changes*

0 to 30 days
removal of debris
necrosis
fibroblast infiltration
30 to 60 days
collagen laid down
60 to 90 days
scar formation

* Peery, T. M., and Miller, F. N.: Pathology. p. 273. Boston, Little, Brown, and Co., 1961.

Signs and Symptoms of Myocardial Infarction

Pain is the most important of symptoms. It may be typical of angina, or it may be atypical, but it always differs from angina in duration, lasting up to several hours or even days. Pain longer than 15 or 20 minutes is almost always pathognomonic of a myocardial infarction.

Other important clues are:
Cerebral
   Psychic: apprehension, anxiety, tension, sense of impending doom
Autonomic nervous system
   Sweating
   Ashen grey color
   Pallor
   Cyanosis
   Cardiovascular shock (pumpless)
Hemodynamic
   Blood pressure (may be normal, or may drop or may even rise)
   Pulsus parvus
   Tachycardia or imperceptible pulse
   Engorgement of venous channels (H. J. reflux is positive)
Cardiac
   (auscultatory)
   Gallop rhythm (atrial and/or ventricular gallop)
   Pericardial friction rub
   Tachycardia
   Arrhythmia
   Changing murmurs or new murmurs
   Fever 24 hours later (necrotic)
Pulmonary
   Acute "asthmatic" wheezes
   Abrupt dyspnea or orthopnea
   Moist basal rales
   Pulmonary edema
   Tachypnea

Gastrointestinal
   "Indigestion"
   "Gallbladder attacks" with vomiting and perspiration

Cardiac Serum Enzymes

Enzyme assays in myocardial disease offer both diagnostic and prognostic aid in the management of heart disease.

Enzyme concentration is measured as enzyme activity and this activity is expressed in terms of the amount of substrate converted. The proposed International Unit of enzyme activity, one micromole of substrate converted per milliliter of fluid assayed per minute (M mole/ml./min.) has not yet been universally accepted; thus the unitage presently is dependent upon the method of assay used.

When cells become damaged, an integral portion of the cellular enzymes exudes through the membrane. The cell must be damaged for this exudation. The amount of enzyme exuded is proportional to the cellular damage and is measured by its content in the serum.

In acute myocardial infarction, enzymes can be found in the serum within 6 to 12 hours. Three of the enzymes used generally are C.P.K., S.G.O.T. and L.D.H. The peak of C.P.K. is reached between the first 18 to 24 hours. The peak of the S.G.O.T. is reached

NORMAL RANGES OF
CARDIAC SERUM ENZYMES

TEST	METHOD	NORMAL RANGE
CPK	Boehringer-Mannheim-IC-V 14992	up to 1 mU/ml.
SGOT	Reitman-Frankel	up to 40 U/ml.
SGPT	Reitman-Frankel	up to 35 U/ml.
LDH	Cabaud-Wroblewski	200-500 U/ml.

between the 2nd and 3rd 24 hours. The peak of L.D.H. occurs about the 3rd day, but an elevated level is maintained for 6 to 7 or more days.

Any reinfarction can be assayed by new peaks or rises in the enzyme levels.

In angina pectoris, the enzyme assays are normal. Heart failure shows elevated S.G.O.T. and S.G.P.T. as a result of hepatic congestion; the enzyme levels will return to normal when this is corrected. In pulmonary embolism, the S.G.P.T. is higher than the S.G.O.T. This is useful as a differential diagnosis between infarction and embolism.

Electrocardiographic Criteria in Myocardial Infarction

Positive Indications of Infarction

1. Q waves of 0.04 second or greater in any lead except aVR
2. Q wave depth greater than 15 per cent in lead I, greater than 20 per cent in lead II, greater than 25 per cent in lead III and greater than 25 per cent of the amplitude of the R wave in leads V_3 to V_6
3. The S-T segment is elevated 1 mm. or more in leads I, II, III, aVL and aVF
4. S-T segment elevation of 4 mm. or greater in V_1 to V_6
5. Cove-plane T waves in leads I, II, III, aVF and V_1 through V_6

Suspicious Findings

1. Arrhythmia
2. Bradycardia
3. Low voltage
4. Presence of Q waves where previously absent

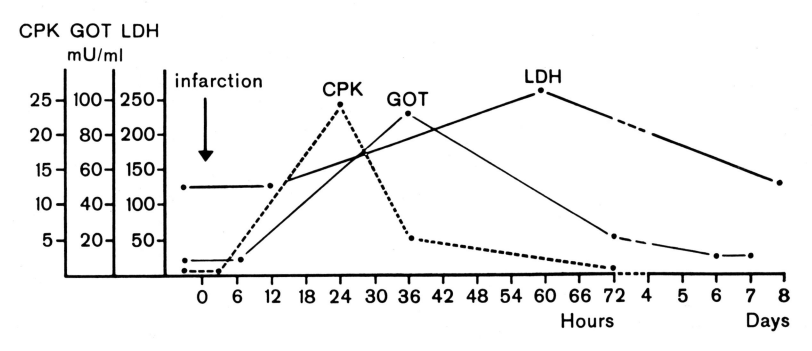

Graph 1. Serum enzymes in acute myocardial infarction. (From: Schmidt, E., and Schmidt, F. W.: Enzymes in medical practice. Biochemical division, C. F. Boehringer & Sons. Mannheim, 1966)

The Necrotic Q Wave
or the Infarction Q Wave

Generally speaking, a Q wave of 0.04 second or greater is considered pathological and denotes necrosis. However, the depth of the Q wave is also important in certain leads. The Q wave depicts an electrical window which looks into the ventricular cavity

Criteria for Abnormal Q Waves

1. Duration 0.04 second or greater in all leads except aVR
2. Lead I: Amplitude of Q wave more than 15 per cent of the amplitude of the R wave
3. Lead II: Amplitude of Q wave more than 20 per cent of the amplitude of the R wave; lead III: amplitude of Q wave more than 25 per cent of the amplitude of the R wave
4. V, or chest, leads: Amplitude of Q wave 25 per cent or more than the amplitude of the R wave
5. The presence of a Q wave in left bundle branch block

Atypical Electrocardiographic Findings

1. S-T segment changes only
2. T wave changes in the absence of Q wave abnormalities — incomplete infarction
3. The development of LBBB or RBBB patterns as the sole manifestation of infarction
   a. Infarction of the interventricular septum
   b. Transient, due to reversible anoxia
   c. Persistent, due to permanent tissue damage (necrotic types)
4. Failure of development of progressive or evolutionary changes
   a. Recording of initial tracing too late

in course of illness; changes missed
   b. Insufficient tracings taken to demonstrate progression during the illness
5. Failure of any detectable ECG changes to develop
   a. Delayed appearance of ECG abnormalities in some cases 7, 14, 21 days
   b. Area of infarction too small to be visualized with conventional leads
   c. Area of infarction located in portion

of heart inaccessible to conventional leads
   d. ECG changes of acute infarction obscured, modified, or completely masked by pre-existing associated, or other ECG abnormalities
   e. Tracings obtained too late in the illness to demonstrate changes (reversion to normal or previous pattern)
   f. Atrial infarction, small posterior

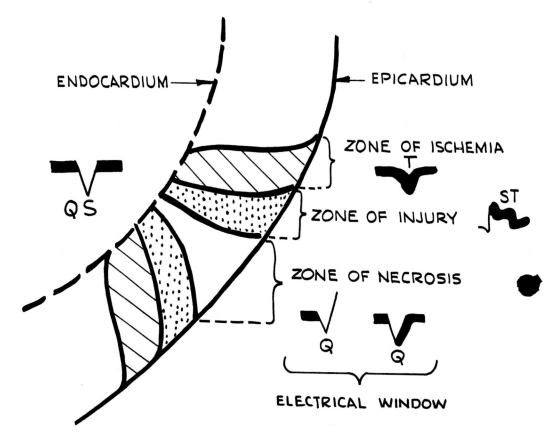

Fig. 11-1. Zones of myocardial infarction.

infarction or high lateral wall infarction

Monophasic Curve of Injury

Very early in the majority of acute myocardial infarctions, the S-T segment forms a typically monophasic curve of injury that may last from several hours to several days. This curve of injury represents subepicardial changes similar to the transudation of potassium on the subepicardial surface of the heart. The monophasic curve of injury is characterized by an elevation of 2 to 4 mm. or more and shows upward convexity. This monophasic curve of injury may be found in any combination of standard leads, unipolar limb leads and in all or a combination of precordial leads. If it is found in one lead only, it represents an acute myocardial infarction of subepicardial nature. Very transitory patterns similar to the monophasic curve of injury are found rarely in acute pericarditis and in acute myocardial ischemia (angina pectoris).

The Electrocardiogram in the Diagnosis of Myocardial Infarction

1. Serial tracings are essential in the recognition of recent or old infarcts. Such tracings may contribute to the knowledge of the size of the lesion as well as the duration, or age of the lesion.

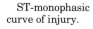
ST-monophasic curve of injury.

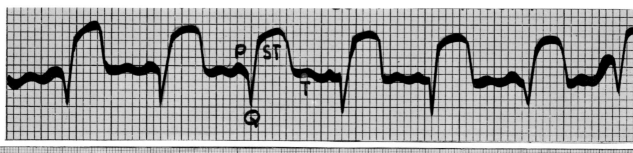

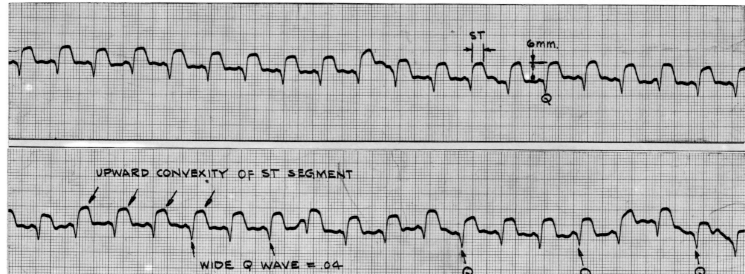

Fig. 11-2. Early acute myocardial infarction (within 24 hours).

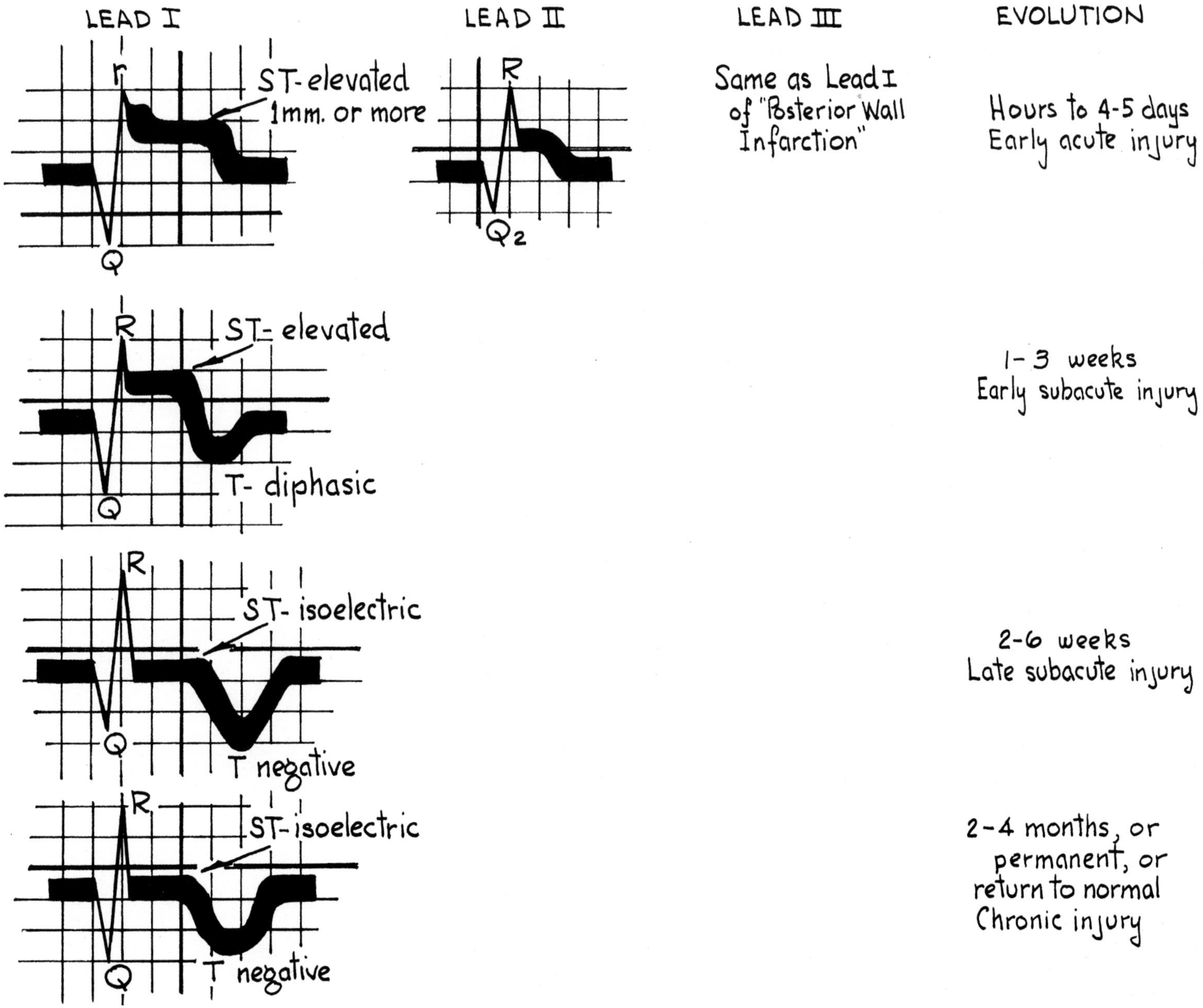

LEAD I	LEAD II	LEAD III	EVOLUTION

LEAD I (top)
r
ST-elevated 1mm. or more
Q

LEAD II (top)
R
Q₂

LEAD III
Same as Lead I of "Posterior Wall Infarction"

EVOLUTION
Hours to 4-5 days
Early acute injury

LEAD I (second)
R
ST-elevated
T-diphasic
Q

EVOLUTION
1-3 weeks
Early subacute injury

LEAD I (third)
R
ST-isoelectric
T negative
Q

EVOLUTION
2-6 weeks
Late subacute injury

LEAD I (fourth)
R
ST-isoelectric
T negative
Q

EVOLUTION
2-4 months, or permanent, or return to normal
Chronic injury

FIG. 11-3. Myocardial infarction, acute anterior wall—Q_1T_1 pattern. Evolutionary stage of anterior wall infarction.

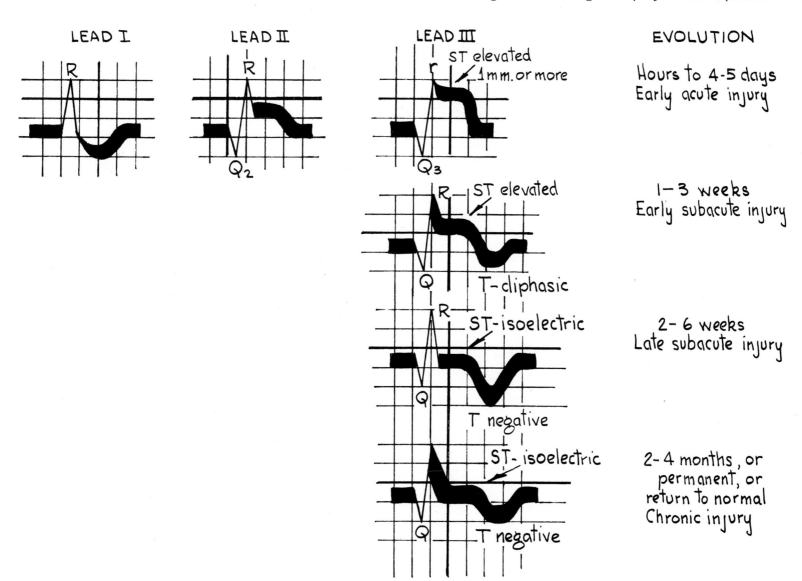

FIG. 11-4. Myocardial infarction, acute posterior wall — Q_3T_3 pattern. Evolutionary stage of a posterior wall infarction.

2. A Q_1 T_1 pattern usually is indicative of anterior wall infarction.

3. A Q_3 T_3 pattern indicates posterior wall infarction.

4. Abnormal Q waves in aVF are found in 60 per cent of posterior wall infarctions.

5. Very low voltage in V_5 and V_6 leads to suspicion of lateral wall involvement.

6. A low T_1 in the presence of a large positive T_3 may be associated with a high lateral wall infarction.

7. Persistence of elevated S-T segments in chest leads is associated with ventricular aneurysm and thrombosis of the left ventricle in 80 per cent of cases.

8. Sudden development of bundle branch block pattern is suggestive of infarction.

9. Sudden onset of Stokes-Adams seizures with heart block may be the first indication of a fresh posterior wall infarction involving the bundle.

10. Ventricular tachycardia almost always heralds infarction.

11. The onset of premature beats, atrial fibrillation, or atrial flutter may also herald infarction.

12. A shift of the axis from left to right axis deviation in the standard leads should lead to suspicion of infarction.

13. Q waves in complete right or left bundle branch block pattern, especially LBBB, raise suspicion of infarction, regardless of size, width or depth.

14. The sudden onset of bradycardia may forbode, or be associated with infarction.

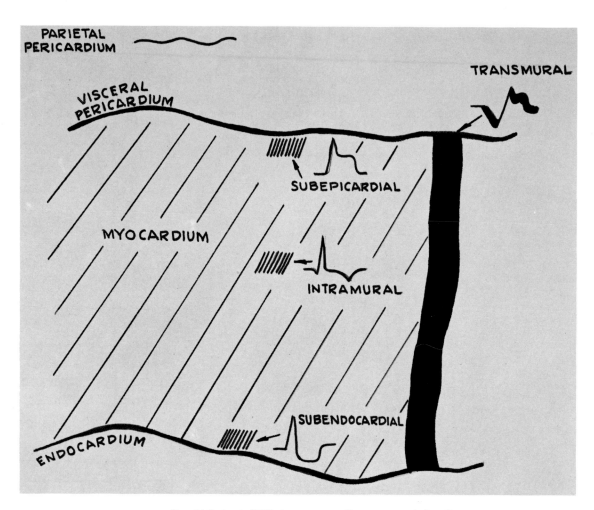

Fig. 11-5. Acute ECG changes according to anatomic location.

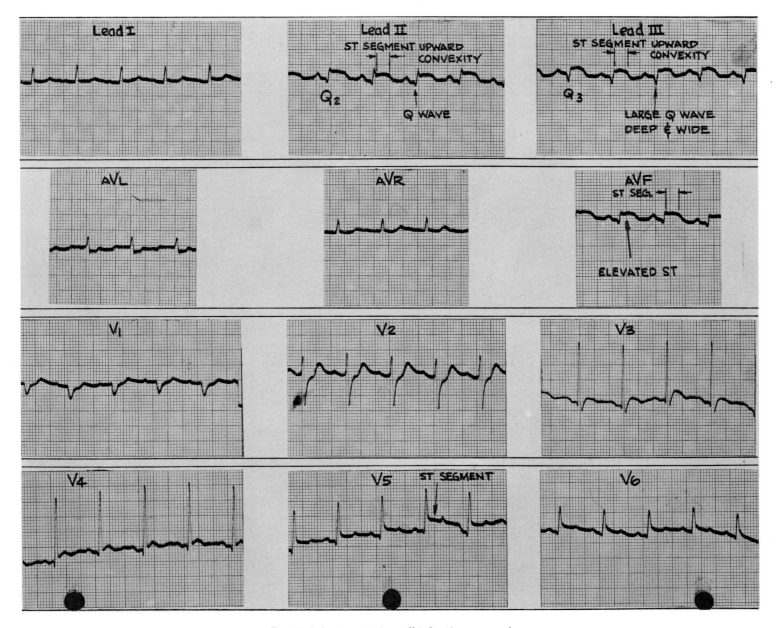

FIG. 11-6. Acute posterior wall infarction, very early: Q_2 and Q_3 pattern.

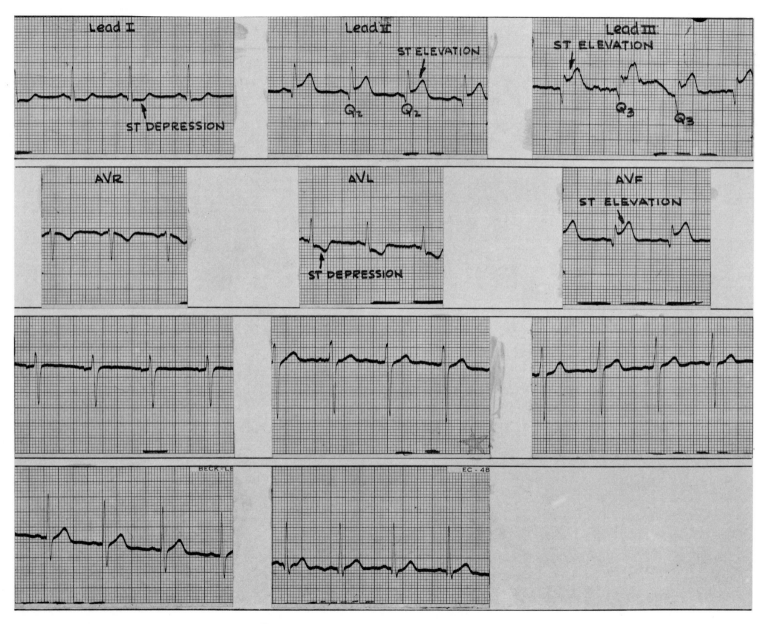

Fig. 11-7. Acute posterior wall infarction. Q_2 and Q_3 pattern.

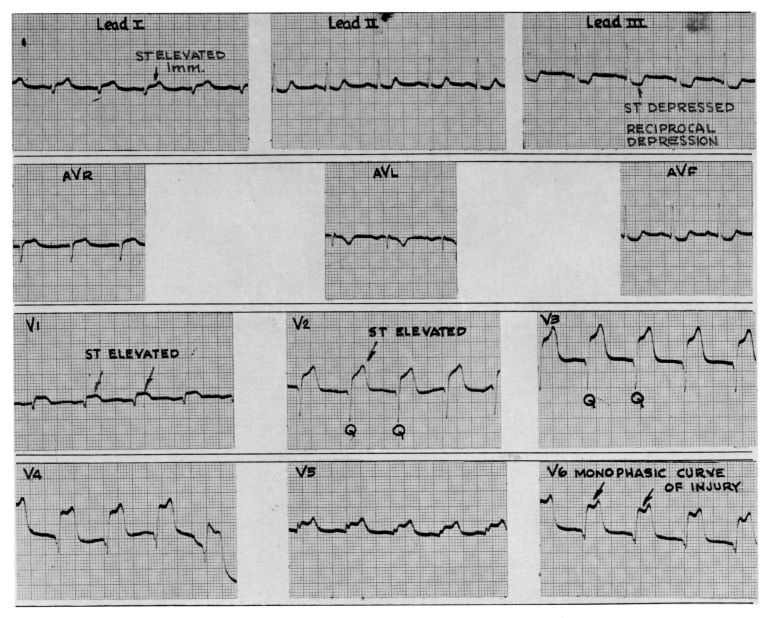

FIG. 11-8. Acute anterior and lateral wall infarction,
extensive. ST elevation in V₃ = 5 mm.

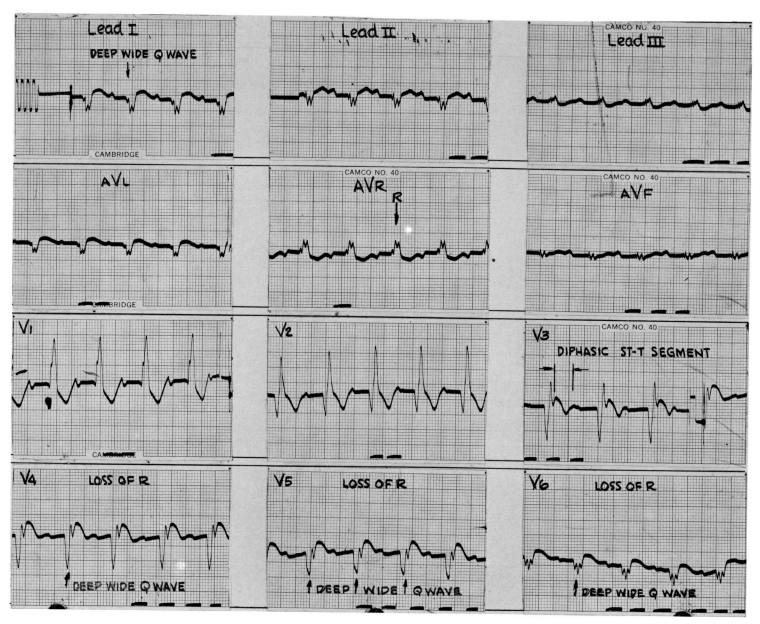

FIG. 11-9. Subacute stage of extensive anterolateral
wall infarction. Cove-plane T waves in V₃.

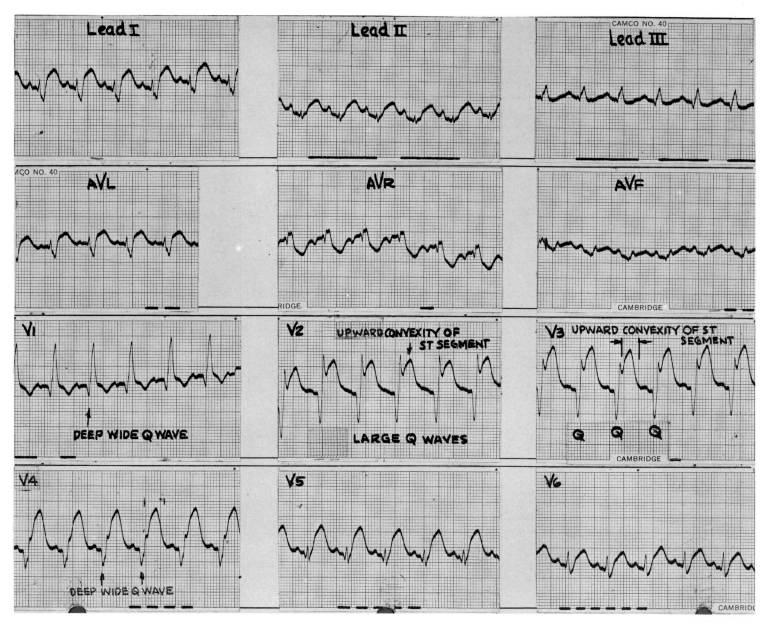

FIG. 11-10. Acute extensive anterior wall infarction.

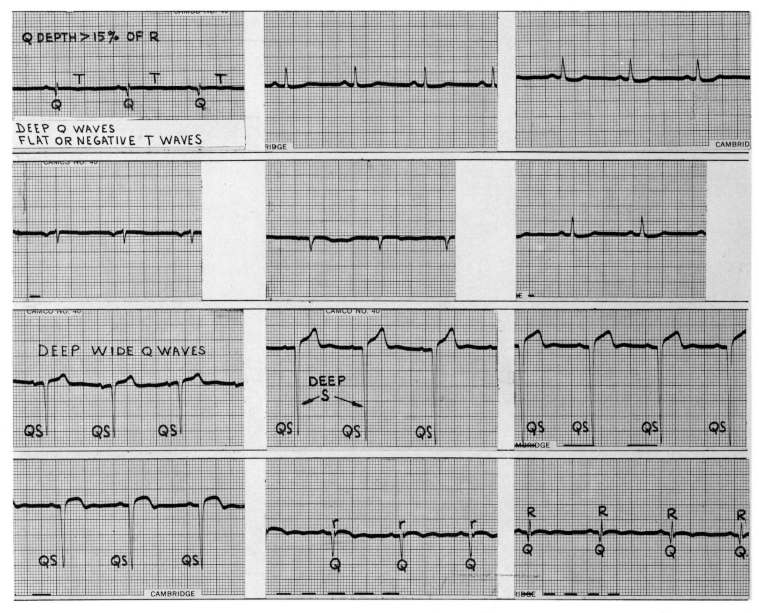

FIG. 11-11. Extensive anterior and lateral wall infarction, chronic: $Q_1 T_1$ pattern.

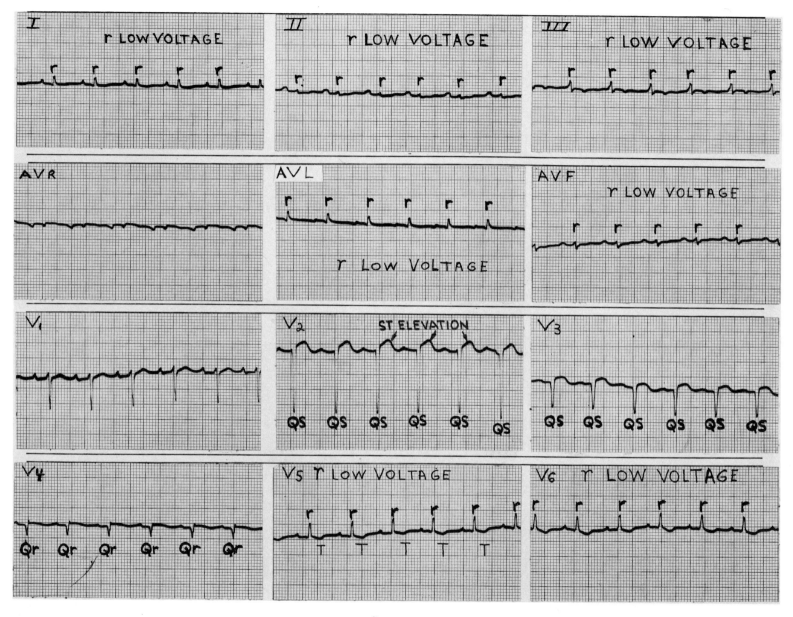

FIG. 11-12. Anteroseptal infarction, subacute stage.
Note low voltage of the r wave in all leads.

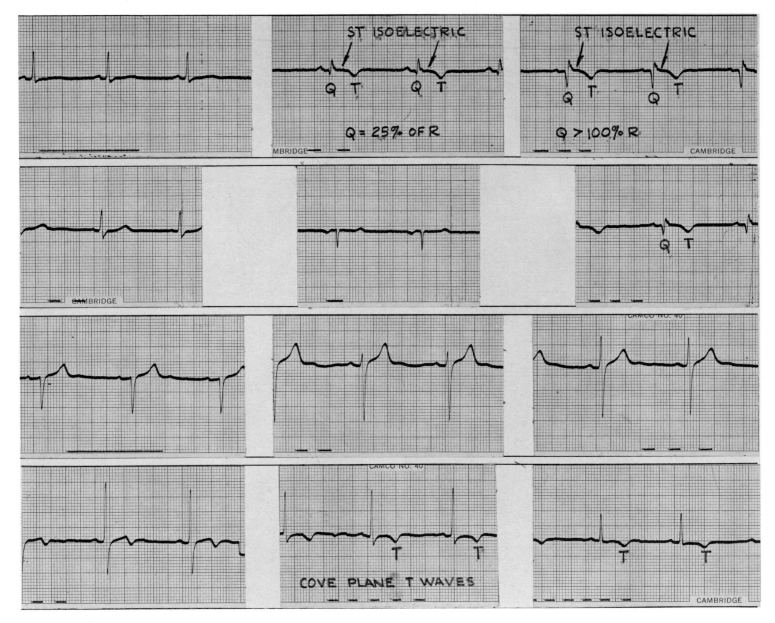

Fig. 11-13. Late subacute posterior wall infarction. Q_3–T_3 pattern.

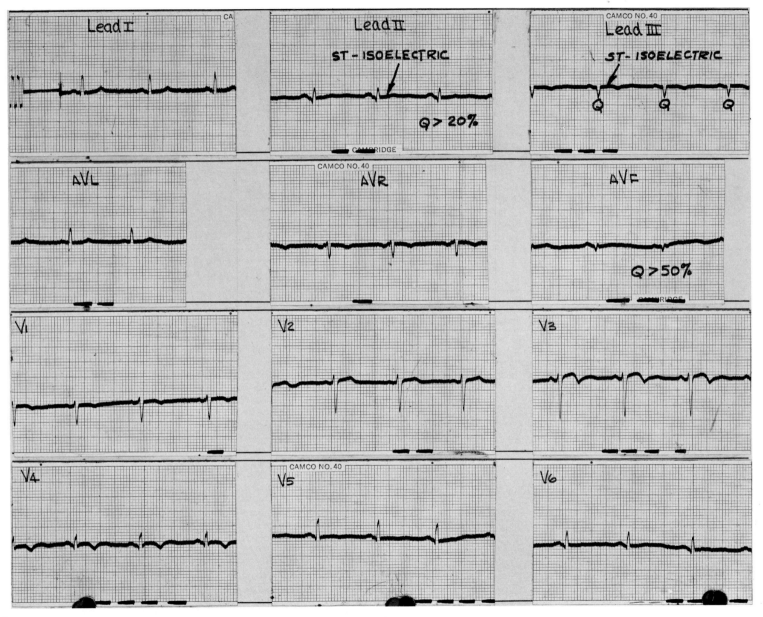

FIG. 11-14. Chronic posterior wall infarction. Q_2Q_3 Pattern. Cove-plane T wave in V_4.

CHAPTER 12

Angina Pectoris

The term *angina* is from the Greek word meaning *to choke*. It describes the clinical symptom of severe chest pain caused by coronary artery disease when the cardiac tissue STARVES, deprived of its oxygen supply. Clinical diagnosis is simple in the classical cases; the "vague" cases can be very atypical. Since the electrocardiogram may be normal, clinical diagnosis is essential. An excellent guide for questioning the patient is the word S-T-A-R-V-E-S.

The Pain of Angina

S   *Sudden* in onset

T   In the *T-zone* — the area across the chest and down along the sternum to the epigastrium, supplied by nerves T_1 to T_5

A   Almost always *anteriorly* located

R   *Radiates* — may extend to the neck, jaw, arms, elbows, wrists and hands, or to the epigastrium

V   *Vagueness* of description of the pain by the patient — a most important symptom. Most patients have extreme difficulty finding something with which to compare the nature or quality of the pain.

E   Induced by *effort, emotion,* or *excitement*

S   *"Stops"* with rest

Questioning the patient with this guide affords a systematic simple plan which is easy to recall.

(See also patterns of S-T ischemic injury.)

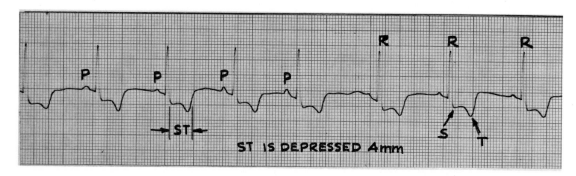

Fig. 12-1. Pattern of ischemia and injury.

Fig. 12-2. Angina, ischemia and injury pattern.

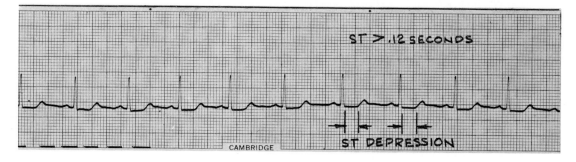

CHAPTER 13

The Master's-Rosenfeld Test
(2-Step Exercise Test)

The Master's-Rosenfeld test is a two-step exercise test, the first step being 9 inches above the floor, the second step 18 inches above the floor. The patient repeatedly and without pause ascends the steps and descends the two steps on the other side.

This is one of many tests used to demonstrate hypoxia or anoxia of heart tissue by S-T changes or other important changes in the electrocardiogram during or after exercise. It is not superior to the other tests but it is simpler to use in office procedures. However, its value is limited because results are affected by the patient's occupation, athletic training etc., and it cannot be used to evaluate patients who are bedridden or invalided.

Electrocardiograms are taken
  at rest
  immediately after the test
  2 minutes after, and six minutes after
    the test

ECG Findings Indicative of
Probable Coronary Artery Disease

Depression of 1.0 to 2 mm. in S-T
Horizontal or sagging S-T segment
(Inversion of T waves, with return to upright T waves after rest, no longer considered significant)

Other ECG Changes After Exercise*†

Arrhythmias (found rarely, and should be documented)
  Paroxysmal atrial tachycardia
  Nodal tachycardia or other nodal rhythm
  Atrial fibrillation
  Multifocal premature ventricular contractions, or two or more successive premature ventricular contractions
  A single episode of ventricular tachycardia
Wolff-Parkinson-White syndrome
Right bundle branch block, complete
Second degree A-V block

Positive Results May Also Be Associated
with the Following Conditions:

Infectious disease
Congestive heart failure
Anemia
Hypothyroidism and hyperthyroidism
Mitral stenosis
Neurocirculatory disorder, in normal patients

* Reported at the American College of Cardiology Conference in Los Angeles, by Dr. James E. Crockett, October 6, 1966.

† From American Heart Journal, 67:830, 1964.

Figures 13-2 to 13-5 demonstrate changes from the cardiogram taken at rest (Fig. 13-2) in cardiograms taken immediately after, 2 minutes after and 6 minutes after a Master's Test.

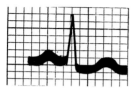

1. **Right-angle S-T segment**

    depression of 1.0 mm or more.

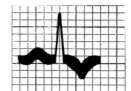 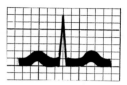

4. **Inverted T waves becoming upright.**

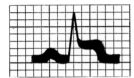

2. **S-T segment elevation.**

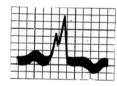

3. **Bundle branch block.**

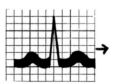 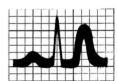

5. **T waves increasing 5 mm or 300% in amplitude, or inverted U waves.**

FIG. 13-1. Some of the positive ECG changes after exercise: (1) Right-angle S-T segment depression of 0.5 mm. or more. (2) S-T segment elevation. (3) Bundle branch block. (4, *left and right*) Inverted T waves, becoming upright. (5, *left and right*) T waves increase 5 mm. or 300 per cent in amplitude, or inverted U waves.

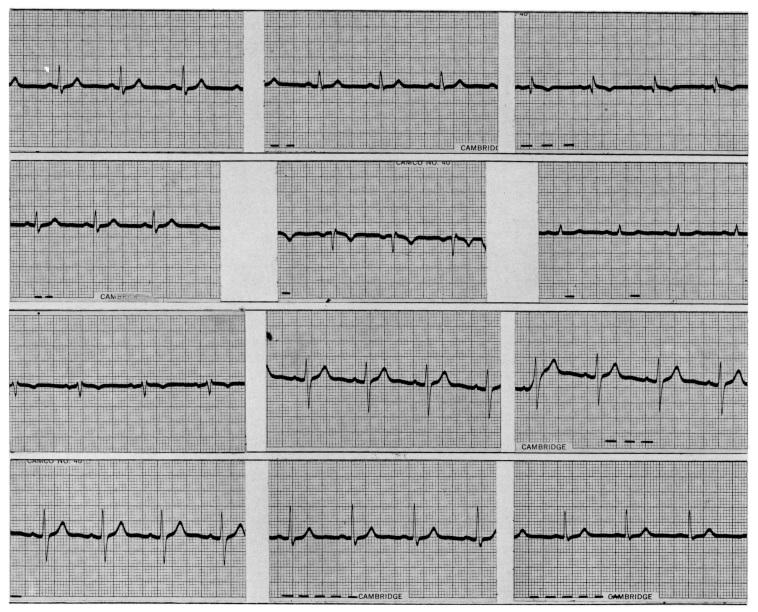

FIG. 13-2. Standard ECG before double Master's test. Resting ECG.

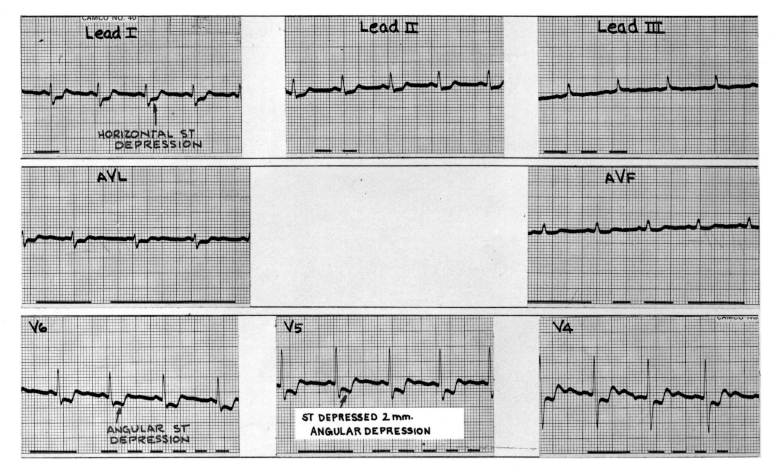

Fig. 13-3. Master's test: ischemia, immediately after exercise.

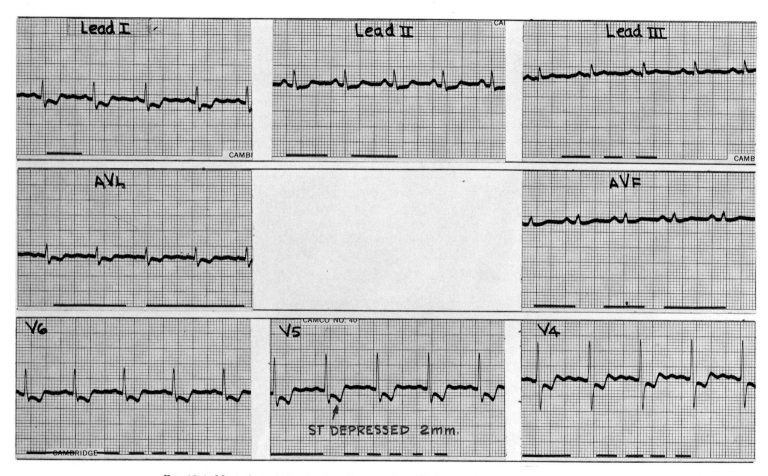

FIG. 13-4. Master's test: 2 minutes after exercise. ST depressed in all leads except lead III and aVF.

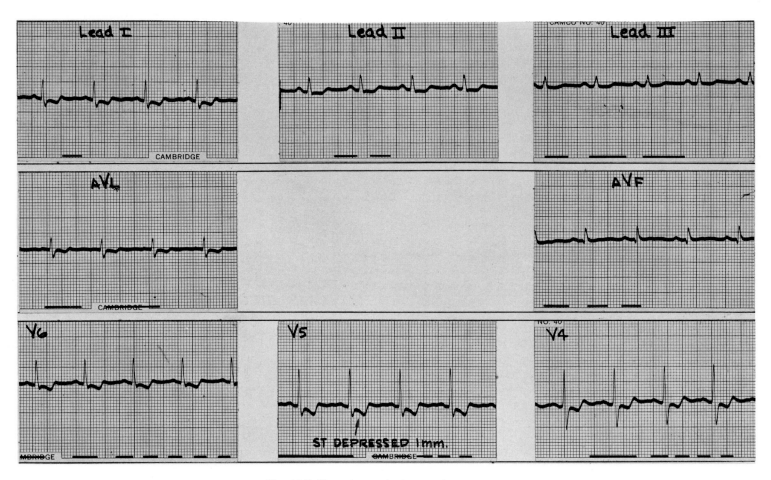

Fig. 13-5. Master's test: 6 minutes after exercise.

CHAPTER 14

Cardiopulmonary Disease:
Cor Pulmonale, Acute, and Chronic

Definition: Cor pulmonale is a specific cardiovascular disease secondary to chronic pulmonary disease and characterized by hypoxia (high pCO_2, low pO_2); loss of pulmonary vascular bed; and right ventricular hypertrophy (increased right ventricular pressure).

Etiologic Factors

Acute Cor Pulmonale
  Embolus from venous system
  Thrombosis of pulmonary artery
  Extrinsic tumor
  Pulmonary embolism (may cause only minimal symptoms or—if massive— sudden death)
Chronic Cor Pulmonale
  Emphysema (most common cause of chronic cor pulmonale)
  Asthma
  Bronchiectasis
  Pulmonary fibrosis due to chronic infection, tuberculosis, chronic bronchitis
  Pneumoconiosis (from inhaled dust or fiber—coal, glass, sand, asbestos, etc.)
  Scleroderma
  Boeck's sarcoidosis
  Schistosomiasis
  Kyphoscoliosis
  (*Text continues on page 129*)

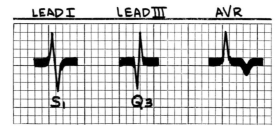

A. McGinn-White pattern (S_1Q_3) is transient, appearing in the first 24 hours. R is upright in aVR and V_1.

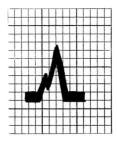

B. Right bundle branch block of sudden onset (2 hours). R is upright in aVR and V_1. (Durant)

FIG. 14-1. (A-D) ECG findings in pulmonary embolism, acute stage. Cor pulmonale.

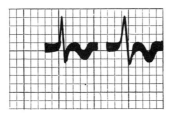

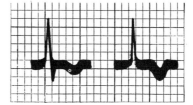

C. T_N pattern: negative T waves in V_1 through V_4. (Wood)

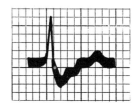

D. Levine pattern (staircase phenomenon) may occur in standard leads and in V_4, V_5, and V_6.

125

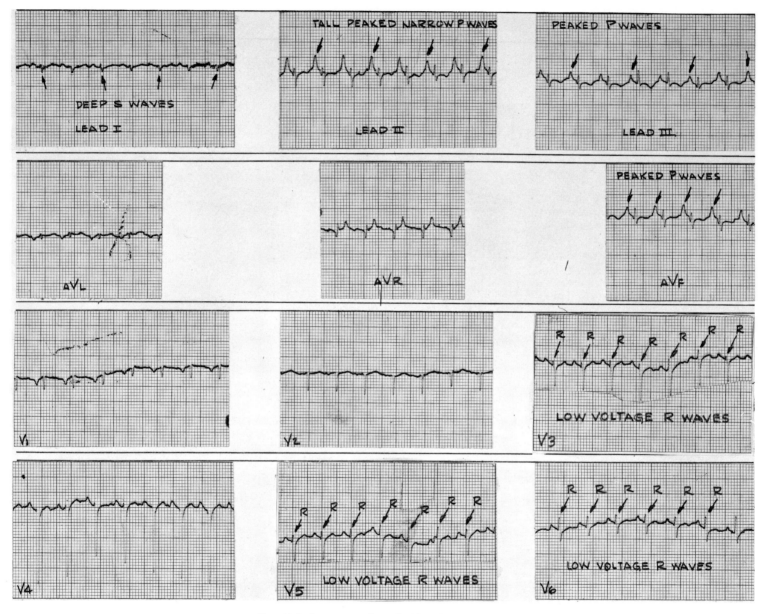

Fig. 14-2. Acute cor pulmonale. Note P_2, P_3, P aVF.

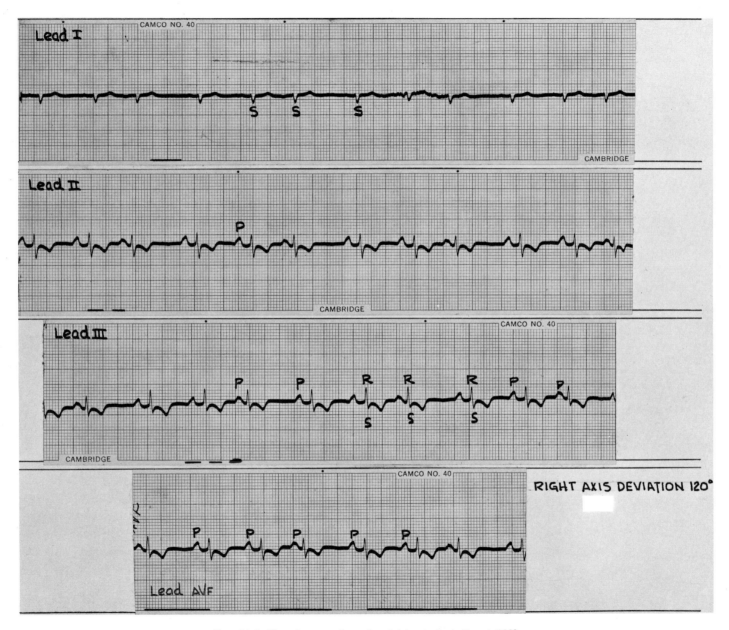

FIG. 14-3. Chronic cor pulmonale: right axis deviation + 120°.

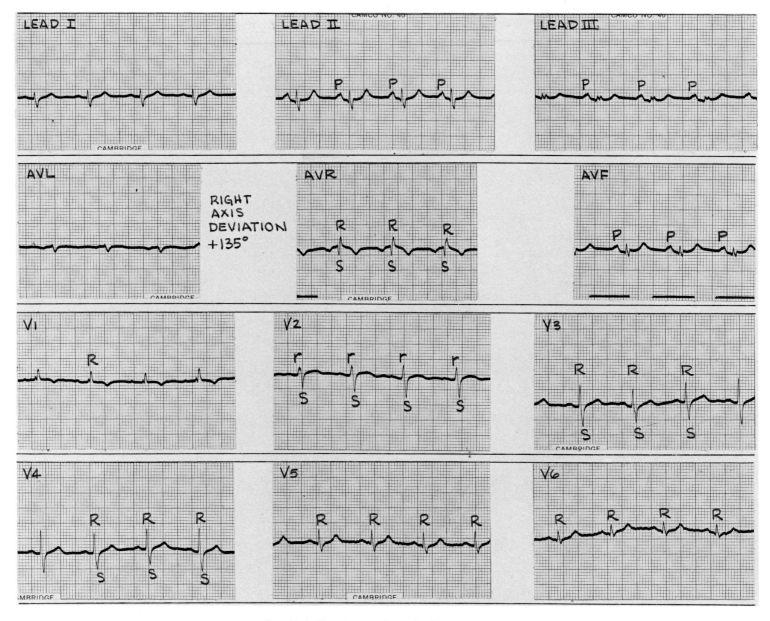

FIG. 14-4. Chronic cor pulmonale, chronic asthma.

Classical Signs of Cor Pulmonale

Sudden pain; cough; dyspnea; cyanosis; engorged neck vessels; wheezes and adventitious breath sounds.

Signs of Pulmonary Embolism

Allen sign: Sudden elevation of temperature, pulse, respiration—associated usually with surgery or active heart disease

F.U.O., in the presence of congestive heart failure or cardiac arrest. (F.U.O. can also be induced by congestive heart failure)

Pathology of Chronic Cor Pulmonale

Loss of elasticity of lung
Reduction of area of vascular bed
Pulmonary hypertension
Right ventricular hypertrophy
Right ventricular failure

ECG Criteria in Acute Cor Pulmonale

S_1Q_3 pattern (McGinn-White pattern)
Sudden peaking or widening of P wave
Staircase effect in S-T segment (Levine pattern)
Sudden onset of right bundle branch block
R taller than 4 mm. in aVR

Pentalogy of Chronic Cor Pulmonale on the ECG

1. Right axis deviation, or tendency toward right axis deviation
2. Peaked P pulmonale waves in leads II, III and aVF, indicative of right auricular hypertrophy (reflection of right ventricular hypertrophy)
3. P wave axis between 70° and 90°
4. Low voltage QRS in precordial leads
5. RS pattern on left side of the chest (V_4, V_5, V_6)

CHAPTER 15

Digitalis and the Electrocardiogram

Action

Digitalis acts directly on the myocardium

Effects*

Therapeutic dosage
  Increases force of systolic contraction
  Shortens duration of systole
  Increases duration of recovery period
  Decreases diastolic size of heart
  Reduces ventricular rate in congestive
    heart failure
  Delays conduction at the A-V node and
    the bundle of His
  Restores sinus rhythm in paroxysmal
    atrial tachycardia
  Encourages diuresis (in congestive heart
    failure)
  Lowers venous pressure (indirectly)

Digitalis has a profound effect on the conduction system (the S-A node and the A-V node) as well as on the heart muscle. As would be expected, each grade of digitalization causes corresponding changes in conduction and rhythmicity and, therefore, in the form of waves and complexes inscribed on the ECG.

*Movitt, E. R.: Digitalis and Other Cardiotonic Drugs. p. 31. ed. 2. New York, Oxford University Press, 1949.

Special Considerations

Digitalis effect as recorded on the electrocardiogram does not indicate dosage, adequacy of amount, or clinical effect.

ECG pattern shows evidence of digitalization for 2 or 3 weeks after the administration of the drug has been discontinued.

Overdigitalization or intoxication produces distinctive changes in the ECG.

Distinctive Manifestations of Digitalis in the ECG

Digitalis Effect

P wave—voltage is reduced; P waves show notching.

A-V conduction—P-R interval is prolonged (drug is implicated if P-R interval becomes shorter when digitalis is discontinued)

RS-T segment—most characteristic in left precordial leads and aVL

S-T segment is depressed; in appearance resembles "strain" pattern

T waves—diphasic; may slope sharply or gradually from negative to positive

Q-T interval—Q-T$_c$ is shortened

Digitalis Toxicity—Digitalis Intoxication

Early Signs or Warnings
  Ventricular extrasystole (one or more p.v.c.)

Premature atrial contraction
Later Manifestations
  Bigeminy
  Nodal rhythm
  Heart block
  Paroxysmal tachycardia
  Atrial fibrillation
  Ventricular tachycardia
  Ventricular fibrillation

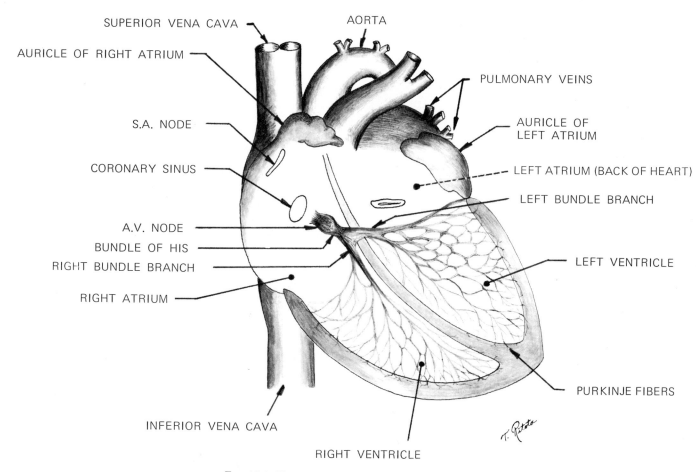

SUPERIOR VENA CAVA

AURICLE OF RIGHT ATRIUM

S.A. NODE

CORONARY SINUS

A.V. NODE

BUNDLE OF HIS

RIGHT BUNDLE BRANCH

RIGHT ATRIUM

INFERIOR VENA CAVA

RIGHT VENTRICLE

AORTA

PULMONARY VEINS

AURICLE OF
LEFT ATRIUM

LEFT ATRIUM (BACK OF HEART)

LEFT BUNDLE BRANCH

LEFT VENTRICLE

PURKINJE FIBERS

FIG. 15-1. Electrical conduction system of the heart.

FIG. 15-2. S-T depression. (*Top*) Concavity (scooped out, or painter's brush effect). (*Bottom*) Angulation: S-T segment forms an angle of 45° with the isoelectric line.

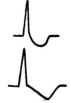

FIG. 15-3. Diphasic T wave.

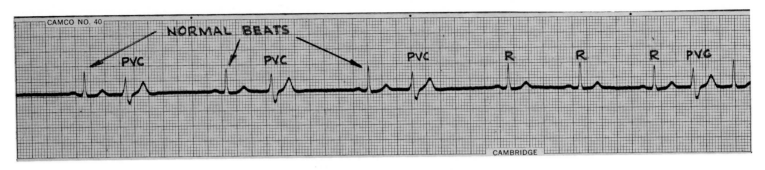

FIG. 15-4. Digitalis toxicity: normal beats are paired
with premature ventricular contractions (bigeminy).

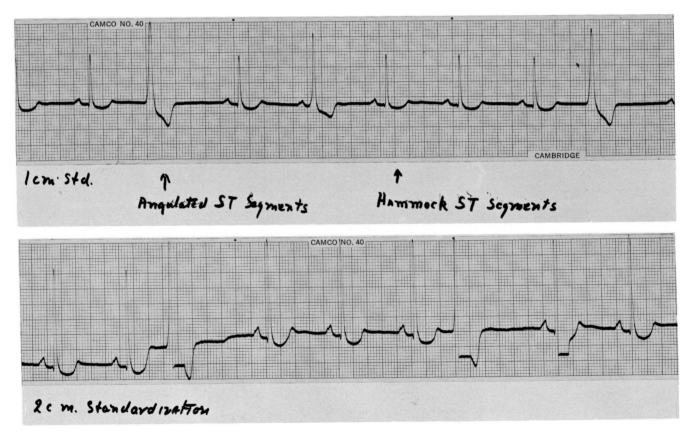

FIG. 15-5. Digitalis effect. S-T segments are angu-
lated or are hammock-shaped. Note how these characteristics are brought out by 2-cm. standardization of
the ECG.

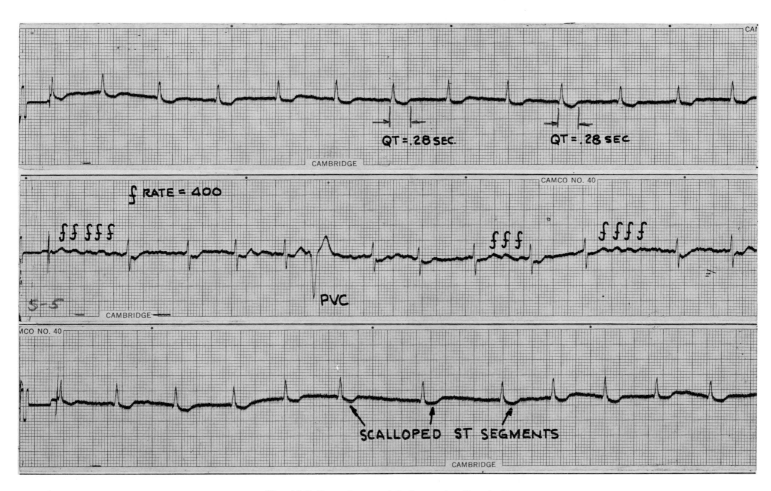

FIG. 15-6. Premature ventricular contractions in the presence of the digitalis effect are suggestive of digitalis intoxication. S-5 or Lewis lead reveals the f waves not seen in Lead I.

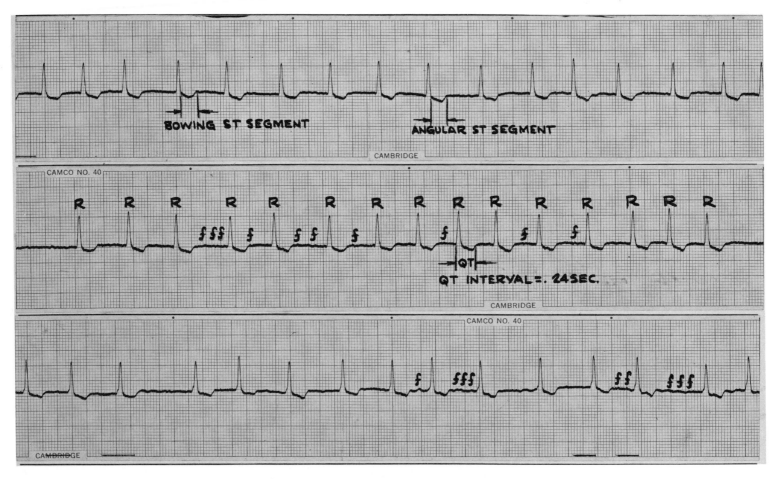

Fig. 15-7. Digitalis effect and atrial fibrillation. Note short Q-T interval (0.24 sec.); digitalis S-T depression; absence of P waves; and irregular R-R intervals.

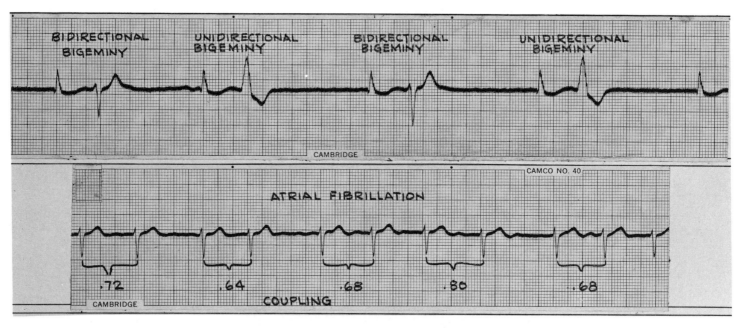

Fig. 15-8. Group beating in atrial fibrillation is suggestive, or may be indicative, of digitalis excess.

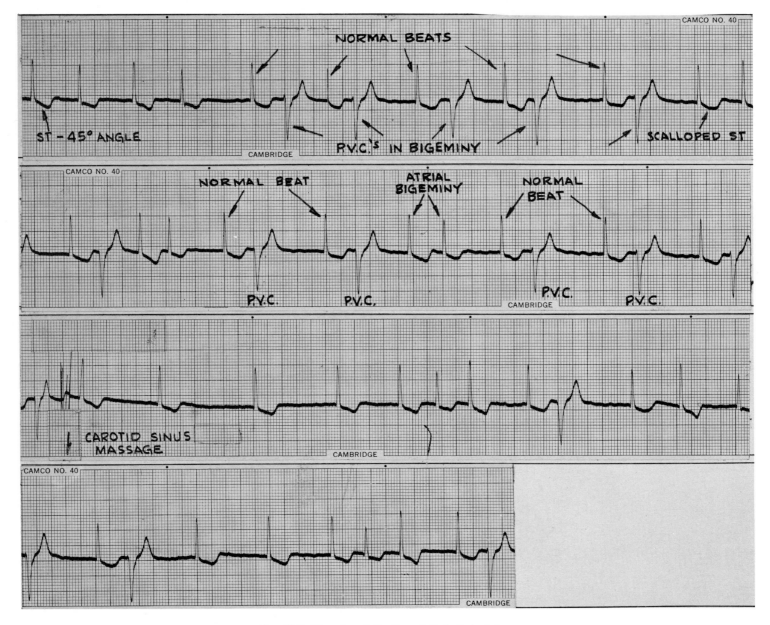

Fig. 15-9. Bigeminy, indicative of digitalis toxicity.

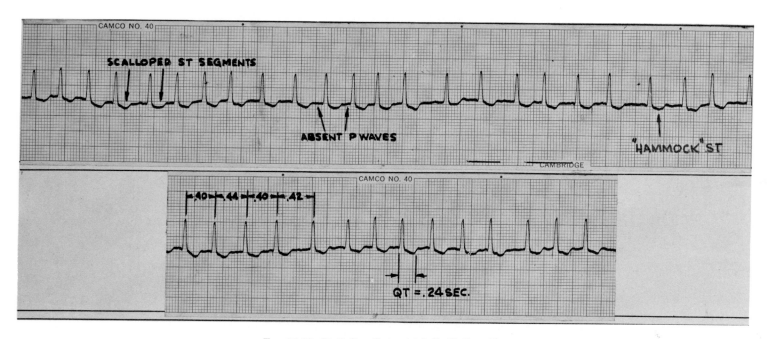

FIG. 15-10. Digitalis effect, atrial fibrillation. Note
irregular ventricular rate and absence of P waves.

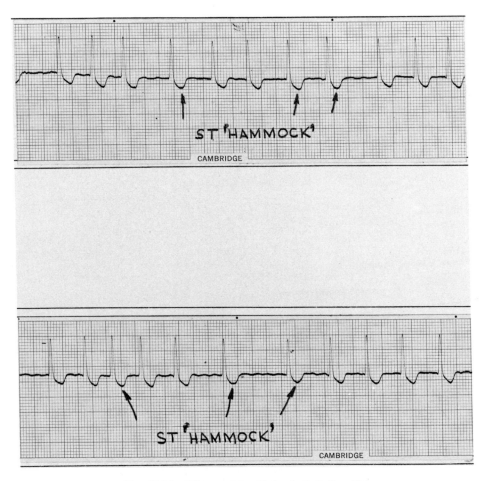

Fig. 15-11. "Hammock" effect of digitalis. Note characteristically short Q-T interval of 0.24 sec.

CHAPTER 16

Electrolytes and the Electrocardiogram

The heart's action is profoundly affected by electrolyte imbalances, especially in regard to potassium and calcium ions. Such effects are reflected in the electrocardiogram, and some are consistent enough to be of diagnostic value.

Hyperkalemia

Causes

Addison's disease
Untreated diabetic acidosis
Acute renal failure
Hemolytic disease
Large number of transfusions
Large oral doses of sat. sol. KI
Hypervolemic shock
Chronic azotemia
Crush syndrome

ECG Criteria*

Intra-atrial block
Low P waves
Prolonged P-R interval (A-V nodal block)
Prolonged QRS (intraventricular block)
Tall, peaked, narrow, "tenting" T waves

Associated Arrhythmias

Sinus bradycardia
Sinus arrhythmia
First degree heart block

* Sampson, J. J.: Am. Heart J., 26:164, 1943.

Nodal rhythm
Idioventricular rhythm
Ventricular tachycardia
Ventricular fibrillation
Ventricular arrest

Hypokalemia

Causes

Starvation
Vomiting
Diarrhea
Familial periodic paralysis
Prolonged diuretic therapy
Excessive digitalis therapy
Excessive use of steroids or corticotropins

ECG Criteria*

Depressed S-T segment
Shortened S-T segment
Slow "take-off" of the S-T segment
Prominent U wave
Prolonged Q-T or Q-U interval

Associated Arrhythmias

Ventricular premature contractions
Atrial tachycardia
Nodal tachycardia
Ventricular tachycardia
Ventricular fibrillation

* Winkler, A. W., Hoff, H. E., and Smith, P. H.: Yale J. Biol. Med., 136:123, 1940.

Hypercalcemia

ECG Criteria*

Short Q-T interval
S-T segment usually absent
Abruptly ascending limb of T wave close to R wave

Hypocalcemia

ECG Criteria*

S-T: isoelectric
       prolonged
Q-T prolonged
Low T waves

* Beck, G. H., and Marriot, H. K.: Am. J. Cardiol., 3:411, 1954.

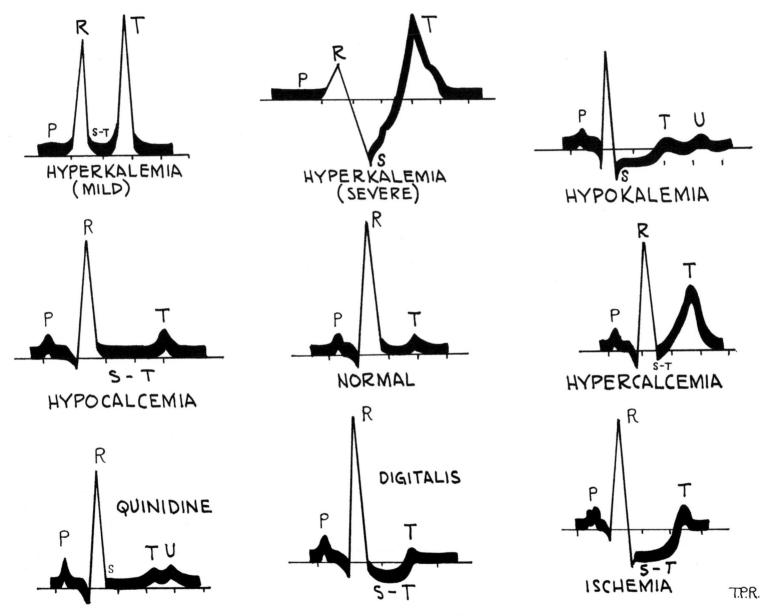

Fig. 16-1. ECG patterns typical of electrolyte imbalances and drug effects, as compared to normal pattern.

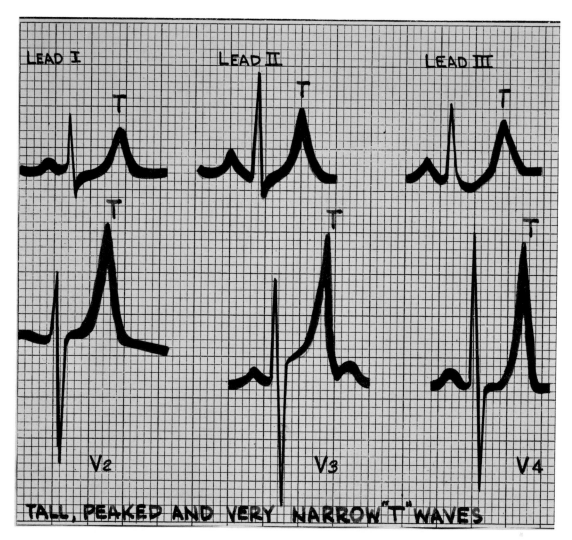

FIG. 16-2. ECG patterns typical of hyperkalemia.

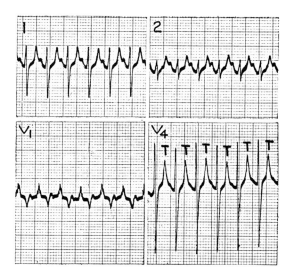

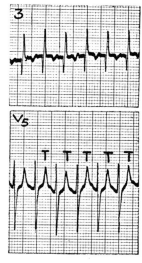

FIG. 16-3. Hyperkalemia: narrow T waves; Q-T interval — 0.20 sec.

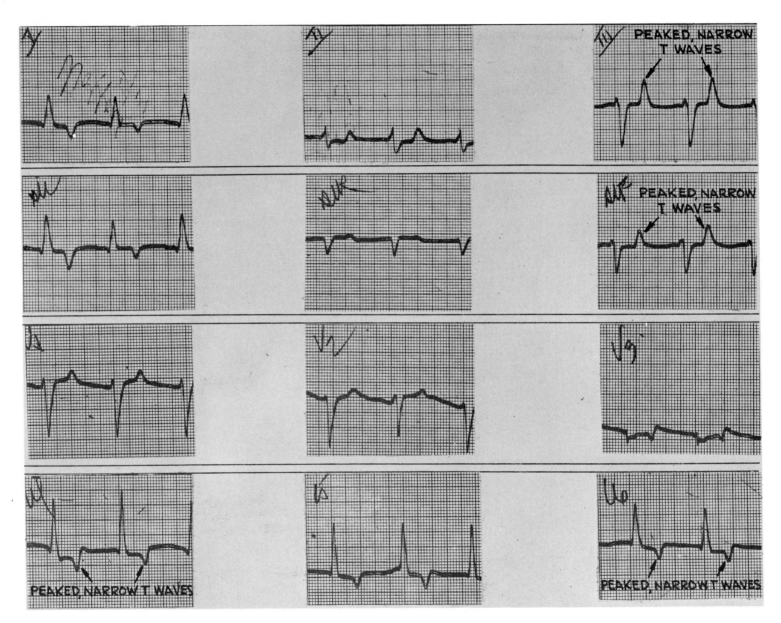

Fig. 16-4. Hyperkalemia. K+ − 9.7 mEq.

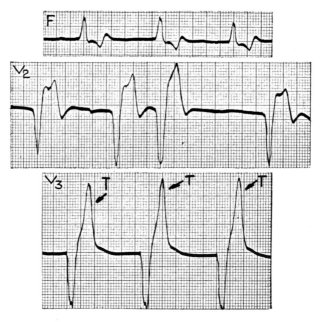

FIG. 16-5. Hyperkalemia. Note tall, peaked potassium T waves.

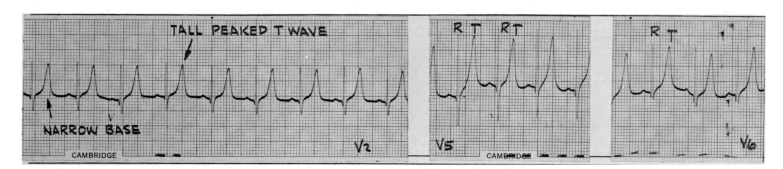

FIG. 16-6. Hyperkalemia. K 6.5 mEq. S-T segment is very short. The T wave has a quick takeoff. The T wave is very narrow at the base.

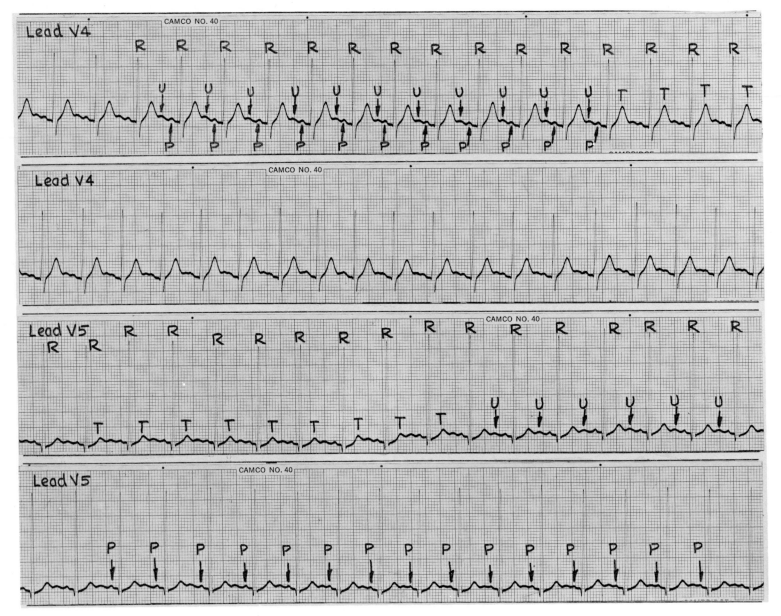

Fig. 16-7. Hypokalemia. S-T depressed in V₅; prominent U waves.

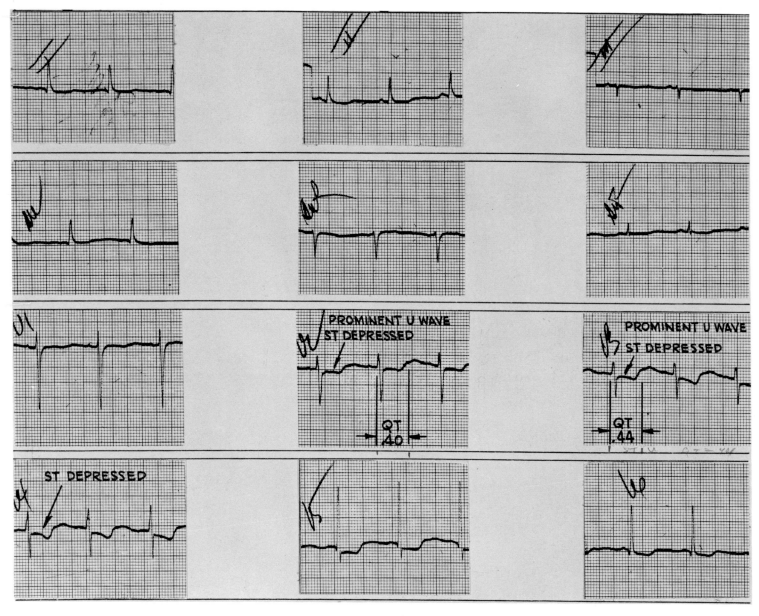

Fig. 16-8. Hypokalemia. K 2.0 mEq. ST depressed, prominent U wave, prolonged QT interval.

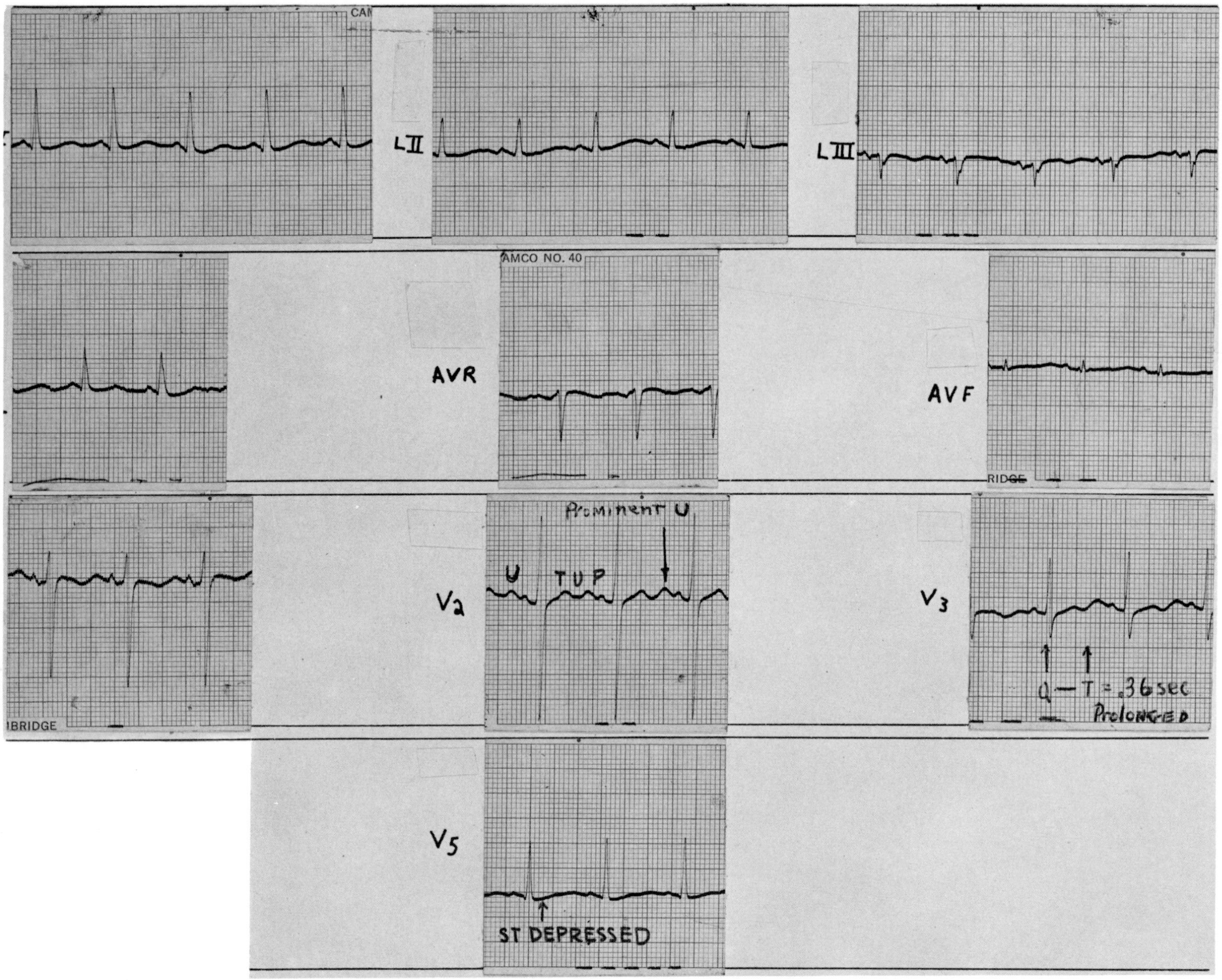

FIG. 16-9. Hypokalemia. 3.0 mEq., post-op colostomy.

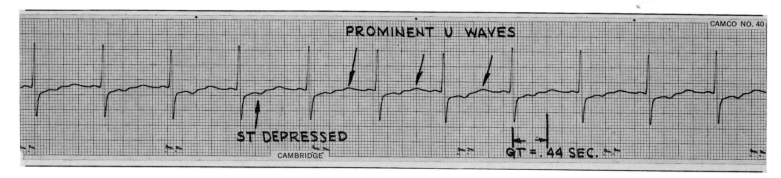

FIG. 16-10. Hypokalemia 3.5 mEq.

CHAPTER 17

Ventricular Tachycardia — Ventricular Flutter — Ventricular Fibrillation — Cardiac Arrest

Ventricular Tachycardia

Definition: Ventricular tachycardia is a rapid, regular rhythm arising from an ectopic focus somewhere in the ventricles, the rate being between 100 and 250. The tachycardia may be paroxysmal or non-paroxysmal in nature. Runs of three or more premature ventricular contractions are considered to be ventricular tachycardia.

Conditions Associated with Ventricular Tachycardia

Digitalis intoxication
Coronary thrombosis, acute

ECG Criteria

1. Onset heralded by a premature ventricular contraction.
2. Ventricular rate of 100 to 250 beats per min.
3. P wave dissociated from QRS
    P wave may be buried
    P wave may follow QRS
4. QRS complex—slurred, notched, 0.12 sec. or more in duration, has all the characteristics of a premature ventricular contraction.

FIG. 17-1 (*Below*) Ventricular tachycardia.

5. Normally conducted PQRS (Dressler beat) may occur.
6. Onset and termination may be abrupt.
7. Rhythm is usually regular, sometimes very slightly irregular.

℞

Procainamide 1,000 mg. in 20 ml. D/W—administer 2 ml. every minute, with ECG monitor.

Lidocaine 50 mg./ml.—give 50 mg. every 15 minutes, to maximum total dose of 300 mg.

Countershock 200 to 300 watt sec.

(*Text continues on page 157*)

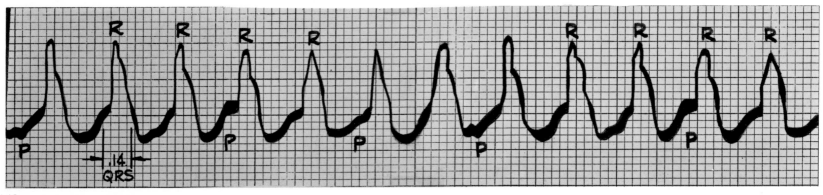

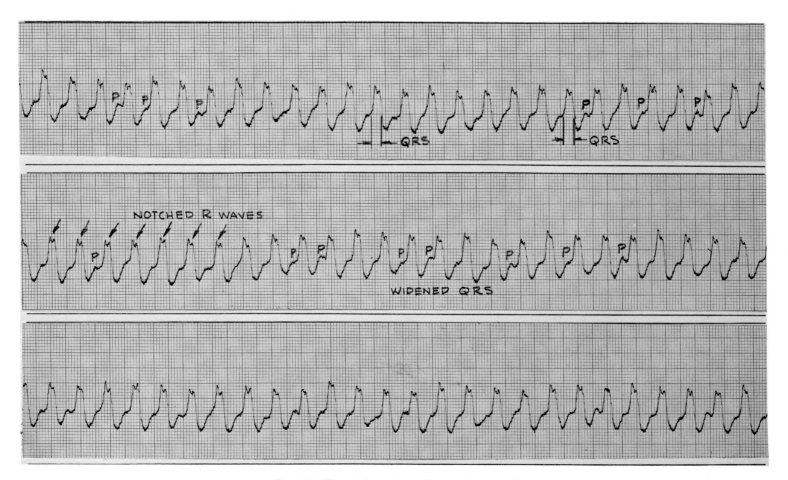

Fig. 17-2. Ventricular tachycardia. Atrial rate—150;
ventricular rate—150. P wave is lost almost completely
in QRS complex.

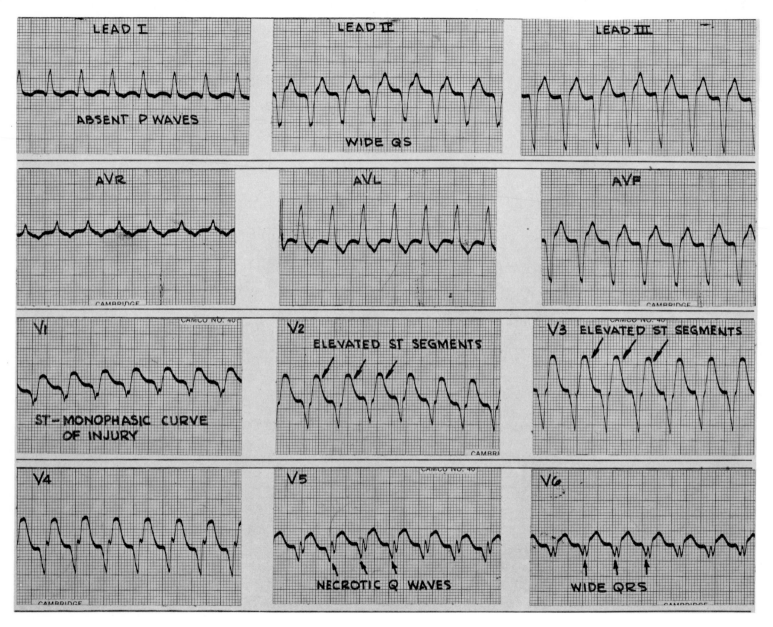

Fig. 17-3. Ventricular tachycardia: extensive acute anterior wall infarction.

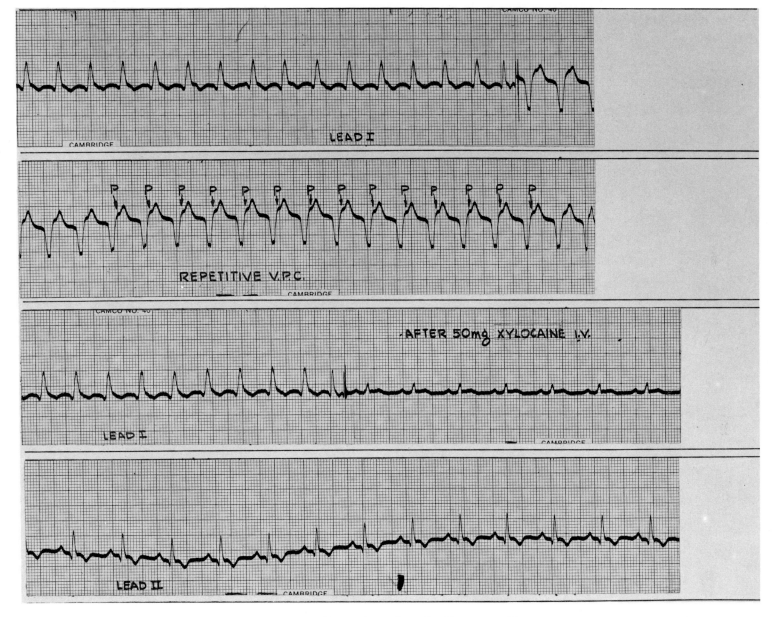

FIG. 17-4. Ventricular tachycardia. Treatment with
lidocaine. Same patient as in Figure 17-3.

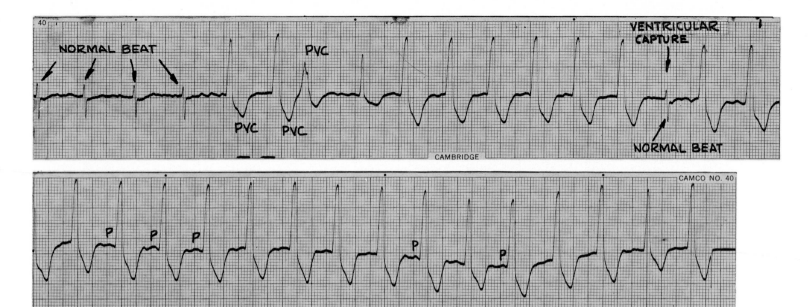

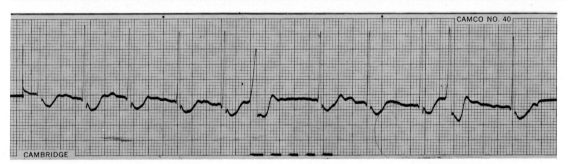

Fig. 17-5. Ventricular tachycardia. Ventricular rate —100. Wide QRS. Normal beats followed by short bursts of 3 PVC's.

Fig. 17-6. (*Bottom*) Ventricular flutter — ventricular tachycardia.

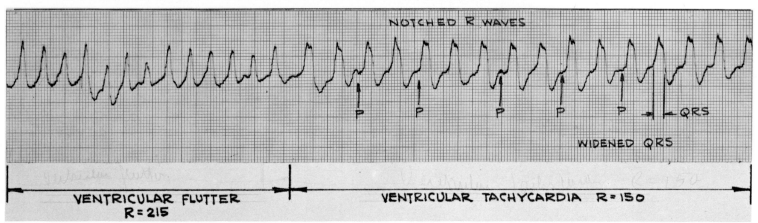

152

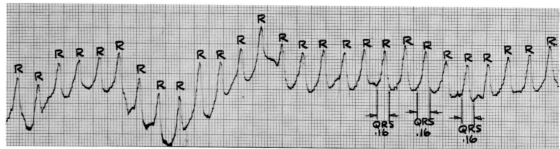

Fig. 17-7. (*Right*) Ventricular tachycardia. Ventricular rate −200; P waves absent.

Fig. 17-8. Conversion of ventricular tachycardia to normal sinus rhythm by use of countershock.

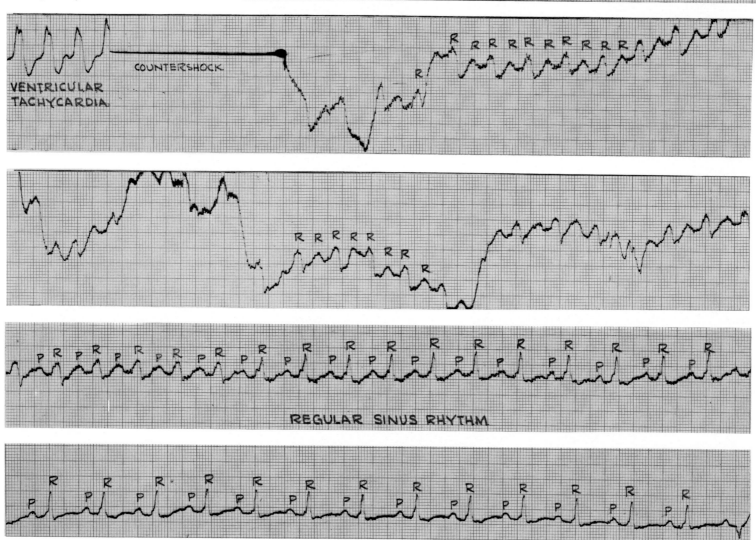

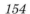
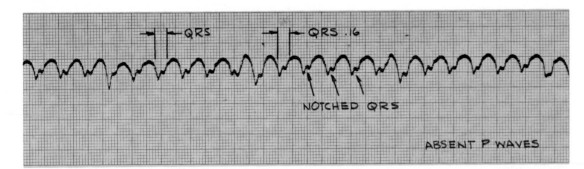

QRS | QRS .16

NOTCHED QRS

ABSENT P WAVES

FIG. 17-9. Ventricular tachycardia: treatment by countershock, and subsequent restoration of regular sinus rhythm.

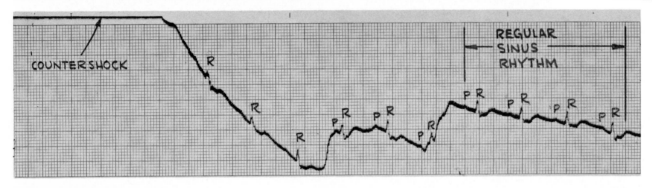

COUNTERSHOCK

REGULAR SINUS RHYTHM

R   R   R   P R   P R   P R   P R   P R   P R   P R

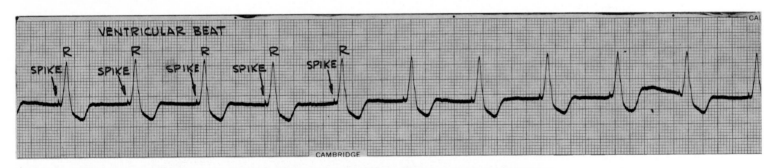

VENTRICULAR BEAT

R   R   R   R   R

SPIKE   SPIKE   SPIKE   SPIKE   SPIKE

CAMBRIDGE

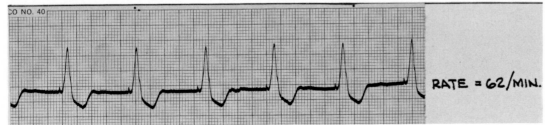

CO NO. 40

RATE = 62/MIN.

FIG. 17-10. Pacemaker ventricular rhythm. Rate—62 per min. Note absence of sinus beat (P wave).

FIG. 17-11. Ventricular tachycardia and ventricular flutter. Upper tracing—severe ventricular fibrillation.

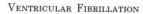

VENTRICULAR FIBRILLATION

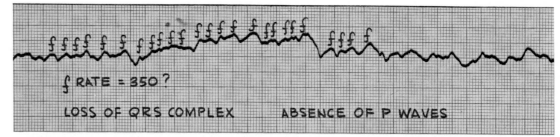

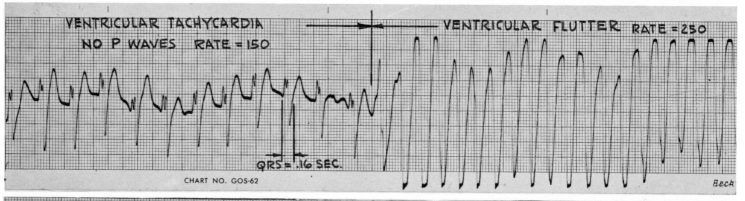

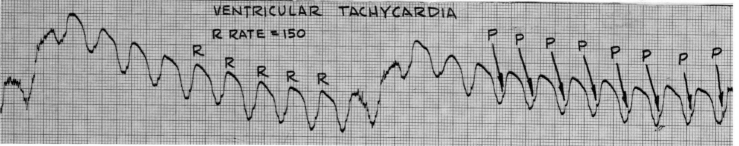

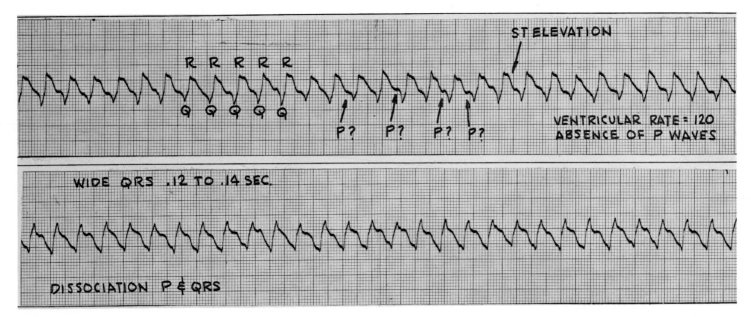

Fig. 17-12. Acute infarction (subepicardial) and ventricular tachycardia.

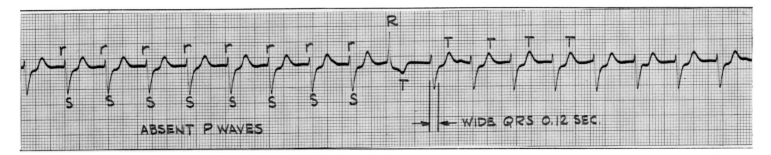

Fig. 17-13. Ventricular tachycardia. Note beat with large R: this is a normally conducted beat, and is known as a Dressler beat. It is pathognomonic of ventricular tachycardia. This is also known as a ventricular capture.

Ventricular Flutter

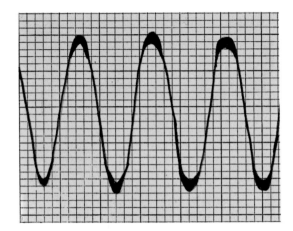

FIGURE 17-14. Ventricular flutter.

Definition: Ventricular flutter is a very rapid beat of ventricular origin, with a rate between 180 and 250 beats per min. It is inscribed as a rhythmic series of bizarre and uniform undulating waves in which there is no resemblance to the normal QRS and no isoelectric interval. Flutter is a severe and advanced form of ventricular tachycardia.

Conditions Associated with Ventricular Flutter

Digitalis intoxication
Coronary thrombosis, acute

ECG Criteria

P waves absent
QRS very wide
T waves absent
Rhythmic and uniform undulation
Isoelectric line absent

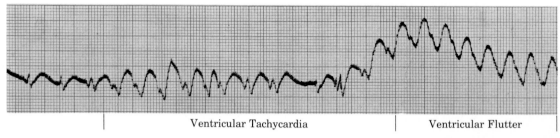

| Ventricular Tachycardia | Ventricular Flutter |

FIG. 17-15. (*Above*) Alternating episodes of ventricular tachycardia and ventricular flutter.

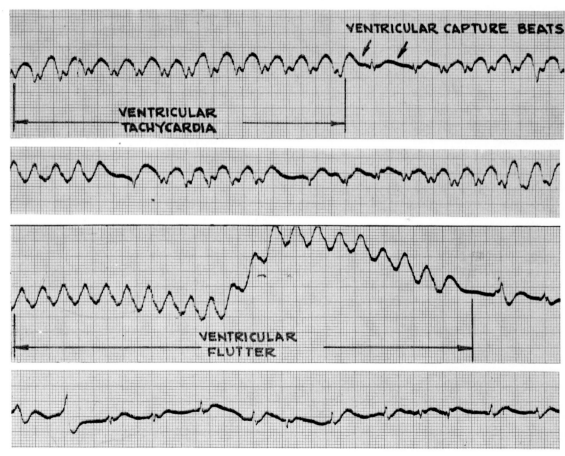

FIG. 17-16. Ventricular tachycardia—ventricular flutter.

Ventricular Fibrillation

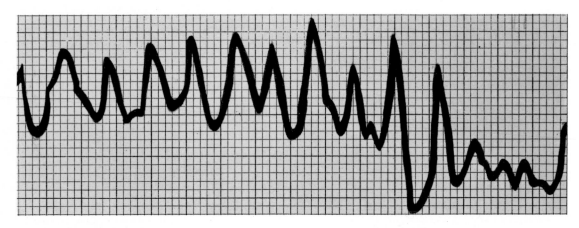

FIGURE 17-17. (Above)

ECG Criteria

Totally irregular undulation
Constant variation in amplitude, width and form
No component of PQRST can be identified
Widely wandering baseline
No isoelectric line
Chaotic rhythm—rate 250-500

FIG. 17-18. (*Below*) Ventricular fibrillation—ventricular flutter.

Definition: Completely incoordinated activity of the muscle fibers, with resultant failure of ventricular contraction. Ventricular fibrillation can be recognized only on the electrocardiogram.

Conditions Associated with Ventricular Fibrillation

Ischemic heart disease
Aortic stenosis
Syphilitic aortic incompetence
Diphtheritic carditis
Complete heart block
Electric shock
Trauma to heart or chest wall
Coronary occlusion
Cardiac surgery
Drug actions
   Digitalis intoxication
   Quinidine excess
   Procaine
   Potassium chloride
   Barium chloride
   Papaverine
   Emetine
   Cyclopropane (anesthesia)

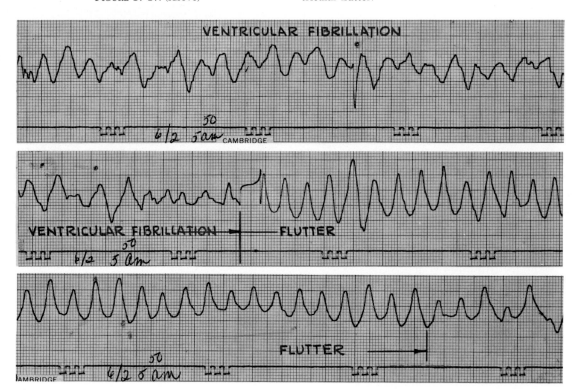

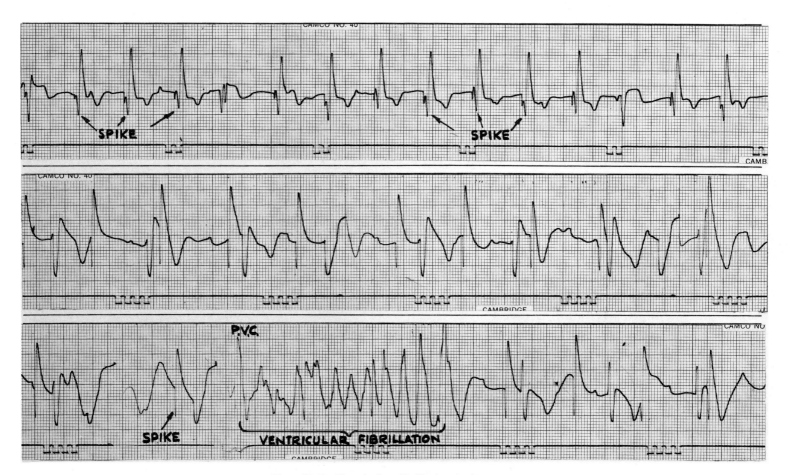

Fɪɢ. 17-19. Ventricular fibrillation in heart controlled by pacemaker. Note that a single premature ventricular contraction precedes episode of ventricular fibrillation. Note spikes of pacemaker.

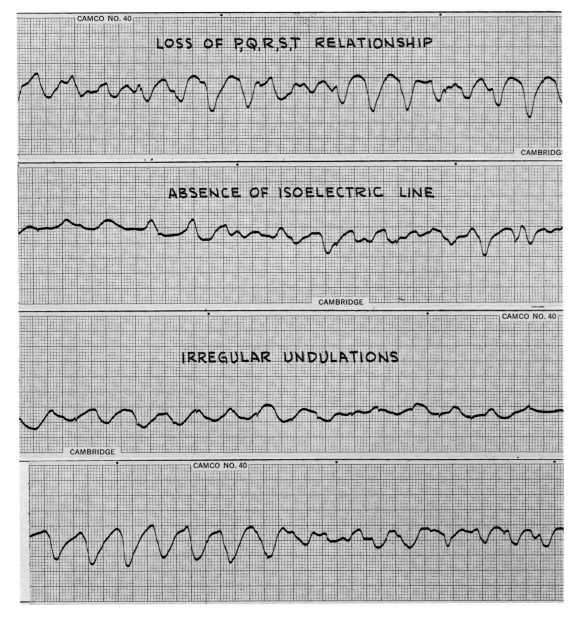

Cardiac Arrest

Factors Related to Cardiac Arrest

Vagus reflex
    may occur during
        pharyngoscopy
        laryngoscopy
        laparoscopy
        rectoscopy
    often associated with hypoxia
Drug actions, particularly after intravenous injection and rapid absorption, of narcotics
    cardiac glycosides
    sympathomimetics
    local anesthetics
    mercurial diuretics
    contrast media
Acute oxygen deficiency, resulting from
    choking
    drowning
    cramps
    myocardial infarction
Severe cardiac arrhythmias, in
    Stokes-Adams syndrome
    accidents involving electric shock
    idiosyncratic reactions
Anaphylactic reactions
    allergies
    penicillins
    anesthesia

Fig. 17-20. Ventricular fibrillation—chaotic rhythm.

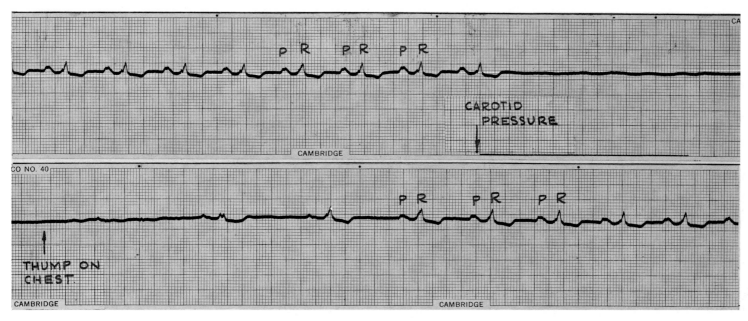

FIG. 17-21. Sinus arrest — asystole.

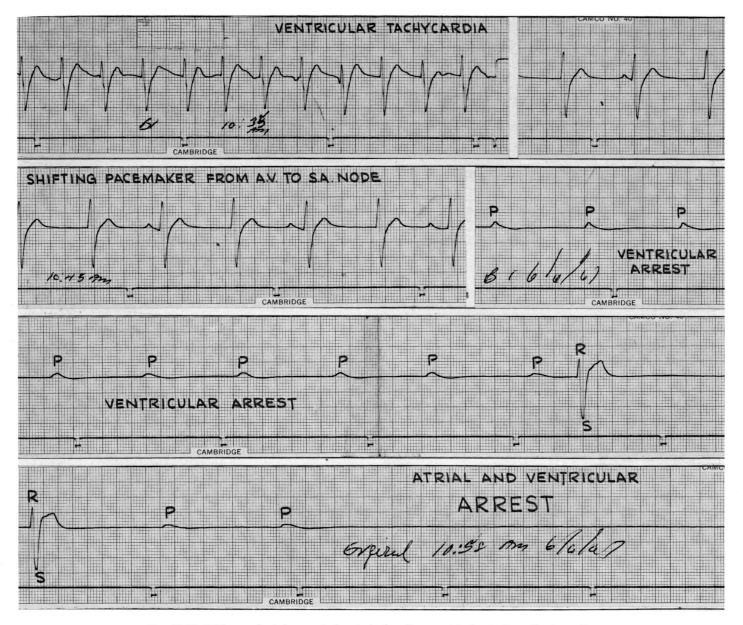

FIG. 17-22. ECG record of changes in heart rhythm from ventricular tachycardia to cardiac standstill. Atrial excitation in lower 2 tracings.

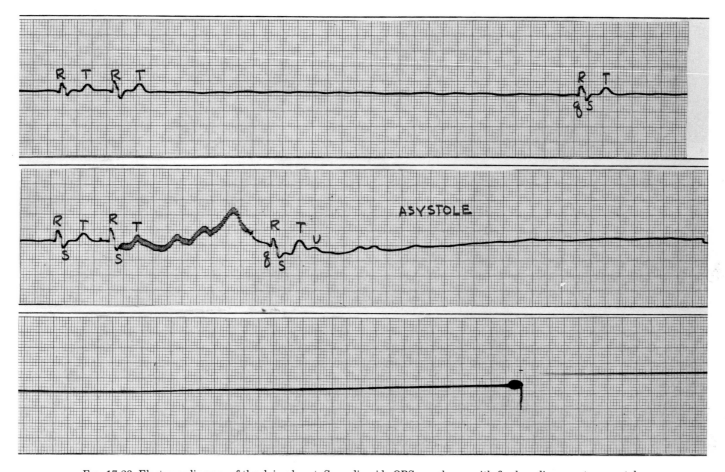

FIG. 17-23. Electrocardiogram of the dying heart. Sporadic wide QRS complexes, with final cardiac arrest or asystole.

INDEX

(Page numbers in
italics indicate
illustrations)

A

Angina pectoris, 118, *118*
  enzyme assay in, 102
Anoxia, of heart tissue, test demonstrating, 119
Arrhythmia(s). See also *heart block* and specific types of arrhythmia.
  atrial, common, 38
  P waves in detection of, 6, *6, 7*
  prolonged QRS in, 11
  sinus, 21. See also *Sinus arrhythmia(s)*.
Atrioventricular block. See *Heart block*.
Atrioventricular nodal conduction, indication of, 7
Atrioventricular node, 82, *82*
  rhythm associated with. See *Nodal rhythm*.
Artifacts, in electrocardiogram tracings, 4, *4*
Asthma, chronic, and chronic cor pulmonale, *128*
  manifestation of, 7, *7*
Atrial arrhythmias, common, 38
Atrial excitation, 5, *5*
Atrial extrasystoles, 40, *40*
Atrial fibrillation, 49, *49-54*
  and digitalis effect, *134, 137*
  and left ventricular hypertrophy, *75*
  criteria for, 50
  group beating in, *135*
Atrial flutter, 38, *39, 46,* 47, *47, 48, 52*
  criteria for, 47
Atrial rhythms, 29-55
Atrial systoles, premature, 40, *41, 42*
Atrial tachycardia, 43, *43, 44,* 45, *45*
A-V node, rhythm associated with. See *Nodal rhythm*.
aVF, and lead I deflection, plotting value of, 28, *28*
Axis, electrical, 22. See also *Electrical axis*.
  deviation, 25
    measurement of, normal, 26
      left or right, 27

B

Bayley triaxial system, 26
Bigeminy, indicating digitalis toxicity, *136*
Block, bundle branch. See *Bundle branch block*.
Block, heart. See *Heart block*.
Bradycardia, physiologic, 33
  sinus, 29, 33, *35, 36*
    criteria for, *35, 36,* 37
    with regular sinus rhythm, *36*
    with sinus arrhythmia, *35, 36*
Bronchitis, manifestation of, 7, *7*
Bundle branch block, 60-69, *60-68*
  complete, S-T segment in, 13
  in exercise test, *120*
  left, complete, *60-65*
    criteria for, *60,* 69
    conditions associated with, 60
  pattern indicating, 11
  right, complete, *67-69*
    criteria for, *66,* 69
    conditions associated with, 60
    of sudden onset, *125*
  T waves in, 14

C

Calcium, excess of, electrocardiographic changes in, 139, *140*
Cardiac. See also *Heart*.
Cardiac arrest, 160, *161-163*
Cardiac rate, determination of, from electrocardiogram, 19
Cardiac rhythms. See *Arrhythmia(s); Sinus rhythm;* etc.
  classification of, 38
Cardiac serum enzymes, in myocardial infarction, 102, *103*
Cardiopulmonary disease, 125-129

INDEX

(Page numbers in *italics* indicate illustrations)

Cholesterol, in myocardial infarction, 101
Coding, lead, 1, 2, *2*
Contraction, ventricular, premature. See *Ventricular systoles, premature.*
Cor pulmonale, 7, *7*, 125-129
  acute, 125, *126*
  chronic, 125, *127*, *128*
  criteria for, 129
  etiologic factors in, 125
  signs of, 129
  T waves in, 14
Coronary artery disease, and myocardial infarction, 101
  tests to detect, 119
Coronary heart disease, recognition of candidate for, 101
Countershock, in ventricular tachycardia, *154*

D

Digitalis, and the electrocardiogram, 130-138, *140*
  excess of, evidence of, *135*
  "hammock" effect of, *138*
  group beating, 135
  T wave in, 14, *15*
  toxicity of, 130, *132*
    bigeminy indicating, *136*
Digitalis effect, 130, *132*
  and atrial fibrillation, 75, *134*, 137
  and left ventricular hypertrophy, *73*, *74*, 75
  and nodal rhythm, *87*
  S-T segment in, 13
  U waves in, *17*
  ventricular contraction in, *133*
Digitalis intoxication, 130
  as cause of nodal rhythm, 83
  early signs of, 130
  evidence of, *133*
  group beating, 135
  premature ventricular systoles as, 59

Dressler beat, in ventricular tachycardia, *156*

E

Einthoven triangle, 1, 23, *23*
Electrical axis, deflection of, in leads I and III, 26, *26*, 27
  deviation of, 24, *25*
    determination of, 25
      by major deflection, 25, *25*, *26*
    left, 25, *25*
    right, 25, *26*
  plotting of, 22-28
Electrical conduction system, of heart, *131*
Electrical field, of heart, and limb leads, 23, *23*
Electrical interference, 4, *4*
Electrical potential, of heart, 24
Electrocardiogram, and digitalis. See *Digitalis.*
Electrocardiogram, artifacts in, 4, *4*
  electrolytes and, 139-147
  indications for, 2
  normal, measurements of components of, *18*
  procedure for taking, 3, *3*
  serial, precautions in taking, 1
  standardization of, 1
Electrocardiographic paper, 1
Electrocardiographic tracings, 1, 4, *4*
Electrode(s), position of, in relation to heart, 22
  precordial, positioning of, 1
Electrolyte(s), and electrocardiogram, 139-147
Electrolyte imbalance, ECG patterns typical of, *140*
  T waves in, 14
Embolism, pulmonary, ECG findings in, *125*
  signs of, 129

Enzymes, cardiac serum, in myocardial infarction, 102, *103*
Exercise, ischemia following, *122*
Exercise test, 2-step, 119-124
Extrasystole(s). See also *Ventricular systoles.*
   atrial, 40, *40*
   nodal, 87
   ventricular, 11

F

Fibrillation, atrial, 49-54. See also *Atrial fibrillation.*
   ventricular, 158, *158.* See also *Ventricular fibrillation.*
Flutter, atrial, 38, *39, 46,* 47, *47, 48,* 52
   criteria for, 47
   ventricular, 157. See also *Ventricular flutter.*

H

Heart. See also *Cardiac.*
Heart, electrical axis of. See *Electrical axis.*
   electrical conduction system of, *131*
   electrical fields of, and limb leads, 23, *23*
   electrical potential of, 24
   leads, facing, 22, *22*
   surface pattern of, 22, *22*
Heart block, 88-94
   complete, 91, *91-94*
     conditions associated with, 91
     criteria for, 91
      idionodal, 91, *92, 93, 94*
      idioventricular, 91
   first degree, 7, *7,* 88, *88, 89*
     conditions associated with, 88
     criteria for, 88

Heart block—(*Cont.*)
   second degree, 88, *90*
     conditions associated with, 91
     criteria for, 91
   third degree, 91, *91-94*
Heart disease, recognition of candidate for, 101
Heart rate, and P-R interval, 7, *7*
   and Q-T intervual, *19*
   and temperature change, 29
Heart tissue, anoxia of, test demonstrating, 119
   hypoxia of, test demonstrating, 119
Hexaxial system, 23, 24
His, bundle of, conduction through branches of, interruption of. See *Bundle branch block.*
Hypercalcemia, 139, *140*
Hyperkalemia, criteria for, 139, *140*
   electrocardiographic changes in, *141-144*
Hypertrophy, ventricular. See *Ventricular hypertrophy.*
Hypocalcemia, criteria for, 139, *140*
Hypokalemia, criteria for, 139, *140*
   electrocardiographic changes in, *145, 146, 147*
Hypoxia, of heart tissue, test demonstrating, 119

I

Infarction, myocardial. See *Myocardial infarction.*
   patterns in, 10, *10*
   Q waves in, 104
   QS pattern in, 8
   S-T segment in, *13*
   subacute, T wave in, *14*
   T waves in, 14, *14, 15*
Interference, electrical, 4, *4*
Intervals. See specific intervals.

INDEX

(Page numbers in *italics* indicate illustrations)

Ischemia, after exercise, *122*
   electrocardiographic changes in, *140*
   myocardial, T waves in, 14, *14*
   S-T segment in, *12*, 13, *13*
   U waves in, 16, *17*

J

J, meaning of, in P-Q-R-S-T-U cycle, 5, *5*

L

Lead(s). See also specific leads.
   code marking of, 1, 2, *2*
   hexaxial system of, 23, *24*
      in plotting major deflection, 28, *28*
   Lewis, *55*
   precordial, 2, *2*
      landmarks for, 3, *3*
      precautions in placing, 1
   standard, 2, *2*
      positioning of, 1
   triaxial system of, 23, *23*
   unipolar, 2, *2*
Lead I, deflections in, 25, *25*, *26*
   plotting of value of, 26, *26*, *27*, 28, *28*
Lead III, deflections in, 25, *25*, *26*
   plotting values of, 26, *26*, *27*
Lead tips, designation of, 1
Levine pattern, in cor pulmonale, *125*
Lewis lead, *55*
Lidocaine, in ventricular tachycardia, *151*
Limb, motion of, as cause of artifact, 4, *4*

M

Master's-Rosenfeld test, 119-124
   ECG, change in, 120

McGinn-White pattern, in cor pulmonale, *125*
Mechanical considerations, 1-4
Metabolic diseases, T waves in, 14
Millivoltage, and standardization of electro-cardiogram, 1
Muscular tremors, as cause of artifact, 4, *4*
Myocardial infarction, 101-117
   acute, early, *105*
   acute anterior wall, *106*, *111*
      and ventricular tachycardia, *150*
      extensive, *113*
   acute anterolateral, *111*, *112*
   acute lateral wall, *111*
   acute posterior wall, *107*
      early, *109*, *110*
   anteroseptal, *115*
   associated with sinus bradycardia, *36*
   chronic anterior wall, *114*
   chronic lateral wall, *114*
   chronic posterior wall, *117*
   criteria for, 102
   diagnosis of, electrocardiogram in, 105
   epidemiology of, 101
   etiology of, 101
   findings in, atypical, 104
      by anatomic location, *108*
      monophasic curve of injury as, 105
   pathologic changes in, 101
   signs of, 102
   subacute posterior wall, *116*
   symptoms of, 102
   T waves in, large, 16
   typical patterns in, *99*
   zones of, *104*
Myocarditis, T waves in, 14

N

Nodal delay, atrioventricular, in heart block, 88

Nodal P waves, *85, 86*
Nodal premature beat, *87*
Nodal rhythm, 82-87
  and digitalis effect, *87*
  and premature ventricular rhythm, *85*
  causes of, 83
  lower, 83, *83*
  middle, 83, *83*
  rate of, 82
  upper, 83, *83*
Normocardia, sinus, 29, *30,* 31

O

Obesity, and coronary heart disease, 101

P

P mitrale, detection of, 7, *7*
P pulmonale, detection of, 7, *7*
P wave(s), 6, *6, 7*
  accentuation of, by Lewis lead, *55*
  amplitude of, 6, *6, 18*
  definition of, 5, *5*
  in nodal rhythm, 82
    forms of, *84*
  in premature ventricular systoles, 56, *57*
  nodal, *85, 86*
  normal, 6, *6*
  notched, *6*
  peaked, *6*
  width of, 6
P wave forms, 7, *7*
P-P interval, in sinus arrhythmia, *32*
P-Q-R-S-T-U cycle, 5-21
  components of, normal measurements and
    ranges of, *18*

P-R interval, 7, *7, 8, 18*
  and heart rate, 7, *7*
  definition of, 5, *5*
  in nodal rhythm, 83, *84*
  normal range of, 7, *7*
  prolonged, in heart block, 88, *88, 89*
P-R segment, definition of, 5, *5*
  junction of, with R wave, *8*
Pacemaker, control of heart with ventricular fibrillation by, *159*
  wandering, in nodal rhythm, 83
Pacemaker fibers, in atrioventricular node,
  82
Pain, of angina pectoris, 118
  of myocardial infarction, 102
Patterns, basic, and portion of heart, 22, *22*
Pericarditis, acute, *95-100*
    and myocardial infarction, *99*
    criteria for, 95
    diagnostic features in, *98*
    early, *95*
    serial tracings in, *100*
  conditions associated with, 95
  S-T segment in, 13
  T waves in, 14
Potassium intoxication, T waves in, 16
Potential, electrical, 24
Pulmonary embolism, ECG findings in, *125*
  signs of, 129

Q

Q wave(s), *18*
  amplitude of, 8, *8*
  definition of, 5, *5*
  in myocardial infarction, 102, 164
  infarction, 104
  necrotic, in myocardial infarction, 104
  normal, 8, *8-10*
  vestigial, 8, *9*

INDEX

(Page numbers in *italics* indicate illustrations)

Q wave(s)—(*Cont.*)
  width of, 8
QR pattern, significance of, *9, 10*
QRS complex, 9, *9, 10*
  in left bundle branch block, 69
QRS interval, *18*
  definition of, 5, *5*
  measurement of, 9, *9*
QRS pattern, and portion of heart, 22, *22*
  prolonged, in arrhythmias, 11
  significance of, *10*, 11
QRS wave, in premature ventricular systoles, 56, *56*
QS patterns, 8, *9*
  and portion of heart, 22, *22*
Q-T interval, 19, *19*
  and heart rate, *19*
  definition of, 5, *5*
  prolonged, 19
  shortened, 19
Quinidine, electrocardiographic changes in, *140*

R

R, definition of, 22
R pattern, *9*
R wave, amplitude of, *18*
  junction of, with P-R segment, *8*
Ramus septi fibrosi, 82
R-R interval, in determination of cardiac rate, 19, *20*
  in sinus arrhythmia, *32*
RS pattern, *10*
  and determination of axis deviation, 28, *28*
  and portion of heart, 22, *22*
Rsr' pattern, *9*
Respiratory movement, as cause of artifact, 4, *4*
Rhythm. See kinds of rhythm.

Rib cage, movement of, as cause of artifact, 4, *4*

S

S, definition of, 22
S-T depression, abnormal, 13
S-T elevation, abnormal, 13
S-T segment, 11, *11-13, 18*
  changes of, in acute pericarditis, *95-100*
  concavity of, *12*, 95
  definition of, 5, *5*
  depression of, types of, 13
  elevation of, in exercise test, 119, *120*
  horizontal, *11*
  in digitalis effect, 130, *132*
  monophasic curve of injury of, in myocardial infarction, 105
  normal limits of, *11*
  variations in, significance of, 13
Segment. See specific segments.
Serial tracings, in diagnosis of myocardial infarction, 105
Serum enzymes, cardiac, in myocardial infarction, 102, *103*
Sinus, regular, and ECG criteria, 29
Sinus arrest, asystole, *161*
Sinus arrhythmia(s), 21, 29-55
  criteria for, 33
  definition of, 29, *32, 33, 35*
  vs. normal rhythm, *32*, 33
  with sinus bradycardia, *35, 36*
Sinus rhythm(s), 29-55
  at various rates, 29, *29*
  irregular, 21
  normal, 29, *29, 30, 31*
  from ventricular tachycardia, *153*
    vs. arrhythmia, *32*, 33
    with sinus bradycardia, *36*
  regular, 20
Sinus tachycardia, 37

ST-T elevation, *14*
Systoles, premature ventricular, 56-59

T

T wave(s), 13, *13, 14, 15, 18*
    abnormal, significance of, 14, *15*
    changes in, in hyperkalemia, *141-144*
        in pericarditis, *95*
    definition of, 5, *5*
    in premature ventricular systoles, *58,* 59
    ischemic, *14*
    large, negative and positive, significance of, 16
    normal limits of, *11, 13*
Tachycardia, atrial, 43, *43, 44, 45*
        criteria in, 45
    sinus, 29, 37, *37, 38*
        and premature ventricular systoles, 58
        criteria for, 37, *38*
    supraventricular, *45*
    ventricular, 148, *148-157.* See also *Ventricular tachycardia.*
Technical considerations, 1-4
Test, exercise, 2-step, 119-124
    Master's-Rosenfeld, 119-124
Tracings, artifacts found in, 4, *4*
    reliable, criteria essential for, 1
Transitional zone pattern, *10*
Triglycerides, in myocardial infarction, 101

U

U wave(s), 16, *16, 17*
    amplitude of, *18*
    definition of, 5, *5*
    negative, 16, *17*
    prominent, 17
    significance of, 16, *17*

V

V leads. See also *Leads.*
    landmarks for, 3, *3*
    marking code for, 2, *2*
Vectors, and electrical potential, 24
Ventricle, left, and electrode pattern indicating, 22, *22*
Ventricular conduction, aberrant, QRS pattern in, 11
Ventricular contractions, premature, *133*
    and nodal rhythm, *85*
Ventricular excitation, tracing of, 5, *5*
Ventricular fibrillation, 158, *158, 159, 160*
    in heart controlled by pacemaker, *159*
    severe, *155*
Ventricular flutter, *152,* 157, *157*
    and ventricular tachycardia, *155*
Ventricular hypertrophy, 70, *70-81*
    and digitalis effect, *75*
    criteria for, 71
    left, 70, *70, 71, 72*
        and atrial fibrillation, *75*
        and digitalis effect, *73, 74*
        causes of, 70
        criteria for, 70
    right, 71, *76-81*
        occurrence of, 71
        precordial leads in, 76, *76, 80*
        S-T segment in, 13
        standard leads in, 71, *76, 80*
        unipolar leads in, 76, *76*
    T waves in, 14
    large, 16
Ventricular musculature, depolarization of, QRS complex recording, 9, *9*
Ventricular rhythm, pacemaker, *154*
Ventricular systoles, premature, 56-59, *56, 57, 58*
    characteristics of, 56, *56*
    clinical significance of, 56
    occurrence of, 59
    P wave in, 56, *57*
    precipitating factors in, 59

INDEX

(Page numbers in *italics* indicate illustrations)

INDEX

(Page numbers in
italics indicate
illustrations)

Ventricular tachycardia, 148, *148-157*
  and acute infarction, *156*
  and myocardial infarction, *150*
  and ventricular flutter, *155, 157*
  conditions associated with, 148
  conversion of, to normal sinus rhythm,
    153
  criteria for, 148
    Dressler beat as, *156*
    QRS pattern in, 11
  treatment of, 148
    lidocaine in, *151*
    with countershock, *154*
Vitamin deficiency, T waves in, 14
Voltage, and standardization of electrocardiogram, 1

W

Waves. See specific waves.